An Informed Decision

An Informed Decision
Understanding Breast Reconstruction

Marilyn Snyder

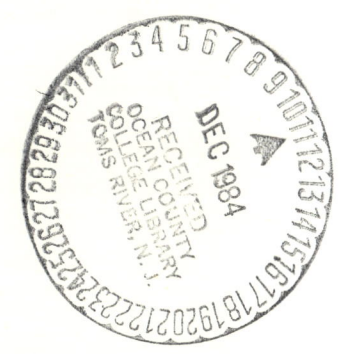

M. Evans and Company, Inc.
New York

Thanks are due to the American Cancer Society and to Rose Kushner, director of the Breast Cancer Advisory Center, for the updated statistics on breast cancer at the beginning of Chapter 1.

The author thanks the following doctors for providing photographs of procedures: Dr. Randolph Guthrie, Jr., for pictures of a Simple Implant Insertion, Simple Implant with Opposite Augmentation, Simple Implant with Opposite Mastopexy, and the Latissimus Dorsi Flap; Dr. Norman Hugo, for pictures of the RAM Flap; and Dr. William Shaw, for pictures of the Gluteus Flap.

Library of Congress Cataloging in Publication Data

Snyder, Marilyn.
   An informed decision.

   Includes index.
   1. Snyder, Marilyn.   2. Mammaplasty—Patients—United States—Biography.   3. Breast—Cancer—Patients—United States—Biography.   I. Title.   II. Title: Understanding breast reconstruction.
RD539.8.S68   1984   362.1'9819059   84-13828

ISBN 0-87131-441-X

Copyright © 1984 by Marilyn Snyder

All rights reserved. No part of this book may be reproduced
or transmitted in any form or by any means without the written
permission of the publisher.

M. Evans and Company, Inc.
216 East 49 Street
New York, New York 10017

Design by James L. McGuire

Manufactured in the United States of America

9 8 7 6 5 4 3 2 1

For Arthur, the children, and Ruth

Contents

	Foreword by Frank E. Gump, M.D.	ix
	Acknowledgments	xi
	Author's Note	xiii
1.	My Story: Alterations and Accommodations	1
2.	Mastectomy and the Altered Ego	5
3.	The Road to Reconstruction	36
4.	Reconstruction at Last	45
5.	Lumpectomy Versus Mastectomy	58
6.	Is Reconstruction for You?	76
7.	A Range of Experience: Monologues	128
8.	Professional Counseling: Ear Lending, Ear Bending	155
9.	Help: How and Where to Get It	168
10.	Questions for the Plastic Surgeon	193
	Index	197

Foreword

Active public participation in health care decisions has been a wholesome change in recent years. Breast cancer has received a tremendous amount of attention because of its high incidence and the controversies surrounding its treatment. While a great deal of informative material has become available in this field, Marilyn Snyder's book breaks new ground. Previous authors have focused on the emotional impact of the diagnosis and the options for treatment. Breast cancer specialists have known for some time that this focus presents an incomplete picture because reconstructive surgery should have an important bearing on the patient's final decision regarding therapy. It truly is the decision of a lifetime, and up-to-date information regarding the amazing advances in reconstructive surgery have not, up to now, been readily available.

This book is admittedly a personal account of someone who has had to deal with breast cancer, but it is far more than that. It provides detailed information covering the many aspects of breast reconstruction, and readers will soon realize that the options in this area are as complex as, as well as more numerous than, those in the primary treatment. Some of the reconstructive methods are so new that physicians are still struggling to better define their limitations and applications. Marilyn Snyder has conducted extensive investigation and interviews, which serve to highlight areas of agreement as well as continuing debate. Her book provides the necessary background information if a woman is to get the most out of a discussion with her doctor. It is complete, up-to-date, and highly readable and will be of tremendous help to women faced with the diagnosis of breast cancer.

Breast reconstruction has had a revolutionary impact in breast cancer treatment. Those of us dealing with this disease now have a valuable, comprehensive source of information about reconstruction to offer our patients. The facts that women require for effective participation in their care are beautifully presented in this most welcome book.

>	Frank E. Gump, M.D.
>	Chief of the Breast Service,
>	Columbia-Presbyterian Medical Center
>	New York

Acknowledgments

I would like to thank the following doctors for their generosity, time and help: David Habif, Francis Symonds, Richard Levine, Jack Weissman, George Hyman, Charles James McGann, Frank Gump, Randolph Guthrie, Norman Hugo, Saul Hoffman, William Shaw, Robert Somers, Jerome Urban, Mary McGrath, and Diane Fink.

For their support and help with this book, my gratitude and thanks to: Charlotte Sheedy, Herb Katz, Linda Cabasin, Tom Cole, Larry Shue, Jane Freeman, Ellen Levine, Judith Daniels, Tom Dunham, François Ilnseher, Gary B. Phillips, Ralph and Judy Schoenstein, Henry Behar, my Kaypro II, Adele Paroni, Felicita Prado, Rose Antonetti, Sue Lucas, Susan Mack, Barbara German, Sondra Bennett, Irene Ladden, Terry Considine, the women in Chapter 7, Linda, Jonathan, and Jennifer Kleet, my family of friends, and my parents, George and Betty Benstock.

Author's Note

The names used in this book are all accurate, with the exception of those of my personal physicians and the women in Chapter 7. Pseudonyms were used in these instances to protect the privacy of the individuals.

This book does not substitute for the medical advice and supervision of your personal physician. No medical therapy should be undertaken except under the direction of a physician.

1

My Story: Alterations and Accommodations

Breast cancer is now killing 36,000 women a year in this country. Early detection is the single most important factor in bringing that number down. Earlier detection is now possible with the help of the process developed by Xerox research: Xeroradiography. It can enable radiologists to identify signs of a malignancy even before a lump develops. The test is simple and takes no longer than other X-ray techniques. This woman is waiting for her doctor to give her the results of her breast cancer test.

The test shows nothing but, for her, everything. Xeroradiography is now in use in many clinics, hospitals, and doctor's offices. It's by no means a cure but it is a means of early detection and, sometimes, a little time can mean a lot.

> —The sound track for a television commercial filmed in New York City in January, 1974

Updated figures on breast cancer in 1984:

1. One in 11 women will develop breast cancer in her lifetime.
2. 115,000 women will develop breast cancer in 1984.
3. 1,000,000 women will be biopsied for suspected breast malignancy in 1984.
4. 38,000 women will lose their lives to breast cancer in 1984.

2 An Informed Decision

I am seated in a large, sunlit waiting room in New York City's Memorial Sloan-Kettering Cancer Center, nervously leafing through a magazine. The lounge is filled with people waiting to see their doctors. The common denominator here is cancer. Everyone in this room either has had cancer or is concerned that he or she might have it. Except me. I am an actress filming a television commercial for a new method of breast cancer detection developed by Xerox Corporation. It is called Xeroradiography, a mammogram or X ray of the breast. There is a camera focused on me for the entire day. My director is assisted by a large crew, Xerox representatives, art directors, writers, and assorted helpers from Needham, Harper, and Steers, the advertising agency designing the campaign for Xerox. Many actresses auditioned, and I feel proud to have gotten the part. The premise of the commercial is that I am a woman who, having detected a breast lump, is anxiously awaiting the results of her Xeroradiogram. In a subsequent scene, her doctor, played by another actor, tells her that the X ray has proved negative, and as the film ends, we see her walk briskly out of the hospital, relieved and smiling.

I did a great deal of research for this part. The hospital even provided me with anonymous inactive breast cancer files. I chose a profile of a woman disconcertingly like myself in age, background, career choice, and family life (a second marriage with young children and stepchildren). Cancer eventually claimed her life, and as I read of the progress of her disease and see the current patients, many of them children on crutches, who are suffering from various forms of cancer, I am struck by an alarming thought. I am the pretender here. Suppose, after playing at this, I am actually back here one day as a real patient. The thought is chilling, and I make a mental note to have my husband, a physician, arrange a mammography appointment for me just to make sure. No sense tempting fate, I tell myself.

It is eleven months later, a blue-skied frosty December afternoon. I'm on my way home to our New York apartment after a busy day of auditions, balancing two bags of groceries for a weekend with my husband, Arthur, and my children, Eric, fourteen, and Nancy, eleven. Fumbling for my keys at the apartment door, I hear a child's quick footsteps and Nancy opens the door. "Mommy, guess what? Nana and Papa are here!" she squeals excitedly. Visits from my parents are a treat for us, but never unannounced. I am surprised but delighted and begin to make mental notes for a festive dinner. Before I can set the groceries down, my mother walks out of the living room to greet me. One look at her face, and I feel a knot of fear forming in my midsection. Beautiful, even in tears, she sobs, "The doctor has found a lump in my breast, darling. We didn't even go home. We drove right to you and Arthur." My father, pale and shaken, is beside her now, his arm around her shoulder, trying to be strong but unable to speak. In a moment I take charge, smothering my own panic, in my need to "mother" my mother, to make her smile. I place a call to Arthur, who immediately arranges an appointment with a colleague, an eminent breast cancer specialist. Since our marriage three years earlier, we have all looked to Arthur for advice and salvation; he is comforting, strong, eternally compassionate. Once again I bless my childhood friend, Norma, for bringing us together.

The doctor tells us the lump must be surgically biopsied. My mother responds in no uncertain terms, "If it's malignant, I don't care how much you have to take off, just get that cancer out of my body!" The procedure confirms our worst fear. My mother has cancer, and a radical mastectomy is performed. The pectoral muscle is removed as well, since the pea-sized tumor is attached to it. The lymph nodes are "clean," free of malignancy; no chemotherapy is prescribed; and the outlook for complete recovery is excellent. When I visit the hospital, I find my father stroking my mother's hand as it rests on the bedcovers. Uncharacteristically demonstrative, he says, "You know, I always thought I loved this little person as much as I could love anybody, but now there's a little bit less of her and I love her even more."

I want to speak but cannot; my mouth feels filled with cotton, stuffed with it as the tops of new pill bottles are with wadding. I struggle to keep my eyes open, at least until I can remember where I am and what I'm doing here. My body feels weighted down; am I tied to this table beneath me? I desperately want water, but am unable to call for it, so weak I can't even turn my head. The only movement I can muster is a roll of the eyes: first upward and then side to side. Where are my glasses? I squint at the clock on the wall. Ten past three? Morning or afternoon? I concentrate hard to jog my memory. A conversation plays back in my head: "If it's benign, you'll be back in your room by noon," my surgeon is saying. "And what if it's not?" I ask. He pats my hand. "That will take a good deal longer, I'm afraid."

Gradually I become aware of two huge yellow-uniformed rear ends, one next to each of my shoulders. I can't see the faces that go with them because I'm still too weak to raise my head. Rear End Number One pokes me in the left shoulder and asks Rear End Number Two, "This is Snyder, isn't it?" Righty replies, "Yeah, the modified mastectomy." I think sleepily, "Ohhhh, I'm sooo disappointed." In my medicated fog, I sense they could have announced that my head was to come off in five minutes and I would still have responded in the same manner. I hear the words, and intellectually it is a profound blow, but emotionally I feel a million miles away from it, still floating in my anesthetic haze. When I come to later in my room, I have the feeling that I have just awakened from a terrible nightmare. And I have.

2

Mastectomy and the Altered Ego

After my mother's mastectomy and as the rate of breast cancer escalated to one in eleven women, it still did not occur to me that I might be seriously at risk. I was in my early forties, in a wonderful marriage with a family of four beautiful teenaged children, and my career as an actress was flourishing. I was convinced that the future had only wonderful things in store for me. My mother had recovered completely, and the specter of cancer had seemed to vanish from our lives. It did not occur to me to visit a breast specialist for checkups. I continued my visits to my gynecologist, who suggested an increase from one to two examinations a year following my mother's illness.

In February of 1980 I accepted a ten-week job at Milwaukee Repertory Theatre in the United States premiere of a wonderful new play from France, *The Workroom*, by Jean-Claude Grumberg. It was an important piece and I had a marvelous role, but leaving my family, my first priority, for ten weeks was not easy for me. However, the play so excited me that on the way home from the audition I had already decided to take the job if it was offered. Nevertheless, I stopped off to get my agent's advice. I ran into his office and blurted out, "Listen, I need to talk to you for a minute."

He smiled, glanced at his watch, and said calmly, "I think I can manage that."

"Well, what do you think?" I asked, short of breath and a little hysterically. "Can I go away to do this play? I haven't been away for work for more than ten days since the kids were born."

He said, "All right, Maggie [my stage name/nickname], answer three questions for me: Do you think it's an important play? Do you love the role? And can your family manage without you?" When I answered affirmatively to all three without any hesitation, he said, "Well, I think we've settled that and we still have thirty seconds left. Would you like to discuss your film career?"

When I raised the issue with my family that night at the dinner table, a silence settled over the little group and then Eric, then eighteen, said, "Listen, I think you should definitely go. I will probably have graduated college by the time you come back, but go ahead." Nancy, fifteen, said, "I am a fragile adolescent and will probably be totally unrecognizable when you return." When I mentioned to my mother-in-law that I was going away to do a play, she said, "It's all your mother's fault. She should have let you do it until you got it out of your system." A few days later, Donald, the elevator man in our apartment building, said, "Mrs. Snyder, I hear you're going away to do a job. How long will you be gone?" "Ten weeks," I replied, marvelling at the speed of communication by gossip. "Ten weeks!" he cried in astonishment. "My God, who's going to take care of them?" When the door opened at our floor, he was still screaming at my back as I ran, key in hand, to the door. "How are they going to eat? Who's going to do their laundry?" Fortunately, Arthur's response was "There's no question but that you must do it. It's an important play and you'll be creating the role for the first time in English. We'll manage and be fine." That's what's so wonderful about Arthur. One of the things, anyway.

Before I left, we decided that Arthur would fly out to visit a few times and that the children would come out at least once.

Actually, we spent every penny that I made flying everyone up and back—including one of my cats to keep me company.

I set about creating mother substitutes in the two weeks before I was to leave: our usual cleaning woman plus someone to help with the cooking three nights a week. Everyone would be taken care of, but I was still very nervous about going. But I went.

As it was, I found that they coped very well without me. I felt a certain ambivalence when I realized that they were actually managing without me. In the last analysis, I felt rather expendable after all. That's a little discomfiting for a mommy—and a wife.

I found, though, that I loved the freedom from responsibility in Milwaukee. It had been eighteen years since I'd catered only to my own needs. I could enjoy my solitary state, secure in the knowledge that I had a loving family back in New York providing stability in my life. It was the perfect combination. I remember feeling slightly guilty about that. But the overriding feeling was pleasure, a delicious self-indulgence.

Two weeks after I arrived, Arthur flew out for his first "conjugal visit," as we termed it. I had planned a wonderfully romantic weekend, having just moved from a hotel room into a compact but comfortable apartment in the same 1930's style hotel overlooking Lake Michigan. It satisfied my nest-building needs, especially after I decorated it with dozens of photographs of everyone in my family, including the pets. That evening, after a romantic dinner at a lakeside restaurant, it was snowing as we walked back to the hotel. It felt so warm and wonderful to be with my husband again, just to have him next to me. Later, as we made love, he touched my right breast. Then I could feel him pull back, almost imperceptibly. He didn't remove his hand, but his touch felt different. He lay back, silent. "What is it?" I asked, even though I knew the answer. He answered softly, "I feel a little something here." He took my finger and put it on my breast, about an inch to the left of the nipple. My left. Stage left, I thought. I felt a little marble-hard bump under the skin. It didn't hurt. It was just suddenly, inexplicably there. How could it have gotten there without my knowing about it? I had not been conscientious about self-examination even after my mother's cancer. I always felt that hers had been the result of estrogen supplements taken to relieve menopausal symptoms. So far as I was concerned, there was no danger to me . . . or so I had convinced myself. Also, I'm not a doomsday person. I don't spend my time worrying about "what if?" Or I didn't then. I had been examined just before I left for Milwaukee. Everything had been fine: no lumps. Now, as I felt this one, the world seemed to turn completely upside down. Even though my mind was saying, "It's nothing, you've probably always had it there," I felt as though I were falling through the floor and down to the bottom of the world . . . as if the earth had opened up and swallowed me. Without a word, I jumped out of bed and ran to the desk phone. It was well after midnight, but I placed a call to a well-known local gynecologist whose name I had been given by a New York relative. His manner was very soothing, and he agreed to see me first thing the next morning. It was a Saturday, but he would open the office for me. Miraculously, Arthur and I both slept soundly, from exhaustion, denial, or both.

After a thorough examination and mammogram, the doctor pronounced the growth harmless, a little cyst, but suggested that if it was still palpable when I returned to New York, I should have it checked again. The mammogram revealed no abnormality. We left relieved and grateful. Eight weeks later, I was back home and the lump was still there.

Arthur and I made an appointment to see my mother's surgeon, Dr. H., on my first Saturday morning home, just to make sure. I didn't even think of the lump that week. I was so delighted to be home with my husband, children, and animals all around me that I spent the days happily cooking their favorite meals, reorganizing the household, and generally wallowing in domesticity. We had a million plans for that Saturday, ending the evening with a tennis party with close friends. Our favorite kind of day together: buzzing around town doing errands, lunch in a quiet restaurant, and so on. The appointment was to be just a brief moment in the whole scheme of the day, my fantasy being that, after examining me, the doctor would say, "Don't be silly. There's nothing to worry about." Instead, while I was still sitting on the examining table, he took my hand in his and said, "I just can't tell, Marilyn. It really has to come out." "You can't?" I asked in disbelief. My voice echoed over and over in my head. This is the wrong script, I thought.

Getting dressed, I realized that I was furious because I felt betrayed by my own body. After all, if I didn't know myself physically, what did I know? And here my body had gone and done something dirty behind my back—or, as Arthur pointed out later, in front of my back. I was livid!

We left the office after we'd discussed all of the possibilities with Dr. H. Later I couldn't believe how calm and detached I had felt at the time, when we'd discussed what measures would be taken if the growth should be malignant. I agreed with Arthur and the surgeon that mastectomy, removal of the breast and lymph nodes, would be the safest measure. Short of that, I felt I'd be gambling with my life. I had several friends who'd had recurrences or died in their efforts to save their breasts by way of lumpectomy, removal of just the tumor and not the entire breast. I just couldn't take that chance. Dr. H. told me immediately that I would be an excellent candidate for breast reconstruction, but at that point my denial of the disease was still so strong that I immediately "shelved" the suggestion in my unconscious. I still believed that all of that intelligent discussion was merely an intellectual exercise.

When I asked if he wanted to see the mammogram from Milwaukee, Dr. H. shrugged. "I see no point. Twenty percent of all malignancies do not show up on mammograms. Your mother's didn't, if you remember. If the cyst were not so hard, I might be able to aspirate it with a needle and examine the fluid for cancer cells. But aspiration won't yield anything in this case and it will only be painful." So much for the mammogram myth.

As we left the office, I remembered my college classmate Betty Rollins's book about her own mastectomy, *First, You Cry,* and I thought, "Well, that's not always so. I didn't." But as we reached the elevator, Arthur put his arms around me. "Are you all right?" he asked gently. Without warning, tears cascaded down my cheeks and I felt as if I were going to dissolve. After a moment or two the tears were replaced by an emotional numbness. My brain felt anesthetized. As we drove home in silence, I looked up as we passed a sign advertising "The New York Death Clinic." In my numbness I thought, "Oh, that's where I must be going." When I turned around to look again, I saw that it was actually "The New York Dental Clinic."

The following Monday, I received a call from a casting director for whom I had worked many times. He wanted to hire me for a day to do screen tests with six young actors being considered for a new role in a daytime television serial. Ordinarily I love to do that sort of thing. It's a treat, a great "muscle stretch." I agreed, thinking it would be a welcome distraction. But what was usually a pleasure was the most trying ordeal imaginable. I could barely get through the day. All I could think of was going to the hospital and that I was in the middle of some dreadful nightmare. The tests took every ounce of stamina and concentration I could muster, and I was absolutely drained by the end of the day. I've often wondered if it showed.

Days passed while I waited for an available hospital bed, and I became a bit more accustomed to the idea of biopsy. I told friends that I had a lump in my breast and it was to be removed for examination. Most people offered positive anecdotes of friends who had gone through the same process. I would listen and respond calmly that I'd only be in the hospital overnight. It was my way of announcing that I would not allow myself to deal with a negative possibility. Trying to pass the time before hospital admission, we visited friends in the country. The husband of the couple whispered as he hugged me good-bye, "Don't worry, everything's going to be fine." I felt enraged, patronized. He didn't know I was going to be fine any more than I knew I was going to be fine. It was the easy thing to say. I told myself that he was trying to comfort me in the only way he knew. It was just that, at that moment, it would have been better to say nothing. So few people can say, "Yes, it may be the worst thing you fear." Only my childhood friend, Norma, said, "Even if it is cancer, you will manage, you will come through it. And then we'll face it together and deal with that reality." It took courage for her to allow me to acknowledge my worst fear. It was lonely carrying that unspoken terror around for two weeks.

I've learned that those who love you want to be included in the bad times as well as the good. They rise to the occasion and feel less impotent if they can help as much as possible. I should have known that about my family. It's just that I always have such difficulty causing that first amount of painful realization. I dreaded telling my parents and sister, but they came through magnificently for me. Traditionally, I was considered the strong one of the family; now I had to allow them to care for me for a change. My stepdaughters were concerned and supportive, and Eric demonstrated his caring with frequent examples of his best football-team bear hugs. Slapping my back, he'd say, "Aw, you're gonna be fine, Ma; c'mon, there's nothing wrong with you." Eric has more denial than I have, or at least as much. Anyway, he comes by it honestly.

Telling my Nancy was particularly hard. One night after dinner I was seated at the kitchen table, she standing with her back to me at the sink. It seemed like the right time, if that were possible. I said, "Honey, I have this little tiny bump in my breast, and the doctor feels that it should be examined since Nana had a problem." I couldn't bring myself to utter the word "cancer"; to verbalize it was to acknowledge the possibility of its presence. Her back stiffened. I said, quickly, "It probably isn't anything bad. We just have to make sure."

She turned and I could see tears on her cheeks. I assumed she needed comforting, so I held out my arms. "Why don't you come over here and sit on my lap? We both need a hug." Unmoving, she looked at me squarely. "First Daddy, then Nana, now you. What about me?" (Her father, my first husband, had undergone a radical mastectomy when he was in his early thirties.)

Her words cut through me like a knife. But, at the same time, I had a tremendous feeling of admiration for this child who had gone immediately to the very heart of the matter: fear for herself. If my mother had told me the same news at Nancy's age, I would have swallowed my rage and done everything to keep her from knowing how furious I was that it represented such a personal risk to me. Nancy said, "It's not that I don't care, Mommy, but I have to be alone to think for a while."

She didn't come out of her room that night and left for school the next morning before I awoke. At 10:00 A.M. the phone rang and I heard her say, "I love you very much, Mommy." My heart swelled for this very special child. Her father is in better health than ever and her grandmother's example is positive: eight years now and no recurrence. I realized how supportive all of my children are, each in their own style. Eric tries so hard to hide his concern, to make me smile. My stepdaughters, Maggie and Katie, are more than generous in their expressions of love. I consider them to be genuinely good, close friends.

I checked into the hospital with my original nuclear unit: my mother, my father, and my sister, Linda. That group still evokes memories of car trips to Florida during school vacations: leaving home while it was still dark to get an early start, the strong smell of gasoline as we made our first "pit stop" on the outskirts of the village. I was a long time out of school, but I still welcomed the comfort of their company, even with the hospital as destination. Of course, Arthur was always nearby. The hospital is his "home away from home." Spending such long days there, he'd always smile at my attempts to urge him home earlier. "Medicine is a jealous mistress," he'd tease. Now that I was a patient, I welcomed his dedication. My little personal fan club followed me around through the admission process, which included the blood tests, chest X rays, and an electrocardiogram. We were very busy trying to keep one another cheerful, insisting that this was a lot of fuss for someone who would be home again in two days. I was assigned a locker and changed into my hospital gown. I have never learned the knack of putting on one of those damn things. I always end up either with it swinging open in the back or not being able to make the ends reach around to tie it. But then, I don't want to be given any more opportunities to master that particular art. I'd rather remain incompetent, thank you.

When I went in for my chest X ray, a cute-looking, curly-haired technician came bustling in. "Hi," he said cheerfully. "How are you?"

"Okay, I guess."

"Are you nervous?"

I grinned. "Well, yeah, a little bit."

"So am I. Isn't it terrible?" I laughed. I never forgot him; he really stuck in my mind, maybe because he made some effort to relax me. Unfortunately, to many of the hospital personnel, the patient becomes just part of the machinery.

My mother was so anxious to have Arthur there with us every minute that she ran up to every distinguished-looking, bearded man in a white coat who walked by my room. After the third case of mistaken identity, she gave up, mortified, but it made us all laugh. Laughter helped a lot that day, so we laughed about everything. We were all so busy hiding the fear. That night, alone in my hospital bed, it didn't occur to me that I might never see my right breast again, or I would have taken pictures.

That evening my anesthesiologist came in to explain his role in the procedure. He extended his hand and said, in heavily accented English, "How do you do. I am your anAthesiologist." Carefully stressing the first *s*, I deliberately repeated the word in question: "Oh, are you going to give me the aneSthesia?" He nodded. "Yes, I give you the anAthesia." I asked a gynecologist friend what it meant if my anesthesiologist couldn't pronounce the name of his specialty correctly. He replied, with a twinkle, not to worry, he'd probably just missed the third year of medical school. As I've said, humor helped—even black humor.

The main terror while waiting to have surgery was not knowing what I would find when I awoke. We had discussed the possibilities. If it was benign, of course, just the lump would be excised; if malignant, the breast as well as the lymph nodes would be removed, a "modified radical." The risk of undergoing general anesthesia twice in a short period made it seem foolhardy to wake me up just to give me the pathology report. I asked Arthur to come to the recovery room and tell me what had been done so that I wouldn't have to lie there and wonder in my anesthetic (excuse me, anAthetic) fog. He later told me that he came in and sat next to me, holding my hand until he was sure I was conscious. Then he gently told me about the mastectomy. He said I appeared to absorb the disappointing news. Tears welled up in my eyes, but I didn't speak. I, on the other hand, have no recollection of his being there at all. Apparently, there is a period during recovery when the patient appears to have complete cognizance but, later, is totally amnestic about that time. Well, that must have been when Arthur told me, because all I can remember is the bulletin from the possessors of those two yellow-robed rear ends.

Immediately after the surgery, Dr. H. called Arthur to report that the lump was actually a tiny malignancy inside a cyst. That explained why it had felt like a cyst on palpation. The axillary, or underarm, lymphatic nodes were removed for examination, as well as all of the breast tissue. Fortunately, the pectoral, or chest, muscle was left intact. So I'd had my modified radical mastectomy.

From the moment I awoke in my room, Arthur never made me feel for one second that I was anything but the most desirable woman in the world—just like my father with my mother. I often wonder what I would have done if I felt he considered me unattractive postsurgery. I had heard of women who felt they had to wear a brassiere to bed because they were convinced that their partners could not tolerate the disfigurement. Perhaps, I thought, it was their own discomfort with their bodies projected onto the men in their lives.

After the surgery it was both comforting and difficult to have my family around me. I needed them desperately, but I couldn't bear their pain. They weren't schooled to disguise it as Arthur had been. Each time I looked into their eyes, I was reminded of that. So I learned to look at their ears or foreheads or make a joke.

During my hospital stay I was a study in manic behavior. I received dozens of bouquets, scores of visitors, colored balloons floating up at my ceiling, stuffed animals of all breeds, books, candy, you name it. As long as I was in the hospital, I was fine. I told myself that it wouldn't make a difference if I didn't let it. Just like my mother: one breast off, and I could deal with it if she had. I was planning to undergo reconstruction as soon as possible, and that would be the end of it. I had it all mapped out. Very neat and tidy.

Well, life doesn't work that way very often. All kinds of subconscious demons were at work from the very beginning. One morning in the hospital, during my usual six-to-eight-wide-awake period, I had a particularly vivid "daymare" (my private label for a daytime nightmare). Daymares, those days, occurred during the hours when it was either too early or too late to phone a friend for help in keeping the worst thoughts away. That particular morning I was lying in bed staring at the blank television screen in its precarious perch near the ceiling. I imagined I could see a little drama being played out on it. I saw myself auditioning for an important part in a Broadway play. There were two producers in the audience, and as I left the theater, I overheard their conversation. One of them said, "Hey, isn't that the woman who had the mastectomy? Maybe we should use her for this part. It calls for character, and she must have more of that now." The other one replied,

"What are you, out of your mind? She could drop dead on us in the middle of the show!" Then I had a vision of my agent, phone to his ear, trying in vain to convince them to hire me anyway.

Aside from the supportive reactions of most of my family and friends, there were those that reflected the terror of individuals for whom the mere mention of cancer evoked hysteria. The prize went to one card from distant relatives: "Horrified to hear of your terrible ordeal. We pray to God you survive." But then there was a dear actor friend, Larry, who took my hand and said, "Maggie, everybody loves you, and nobody ever loved you for your right breast." That was exactly what I had to hear. A memorable letter from my college friend Scottie read: "Remember on your 'down days' that the reason for that operation is to make you well. The alternative is much worse." Such messages helped immeasurably to keep my priorities in order.

The day I was due to check out of the hospital, I woke at my usual 6 A.M., terrified at the thought of leaving that cocoon where abnormal was normal. I kept thinking of my old definition of human behavior: "Normal is what your friends are doing." Well, my in-hospital social circle was definitely not the same as that at home. That morning I was acutely aware of the difference. It was still too early to use my phone as therapy, but I remembered the tape recorder I had brought with me. I have always been a notoriously poor correspondent, and taping was an excellent way of sending a "talking" letter. I turned it on and for one hour recorded all of my terror. It helped enormously to calm me, and I resolved to make such "talks" a daily part of my routine. I hoped that it would save not only the ears of my family but my sanity as well.

Just before I left the hospital, our Portuguese cleaning lady, Guillermina, telephoned me.

"Hello, Mrs. Sny-ner?"

"Oh, hello, Guillermina, how are you?"

"No, how are *you*, Mrs. Sny-ner, how are *you?*"

"Oh, I'm fine, really."

"Nooooo."

"Yes, Guillermina, you don't have to worry about me. I really am feeling okay."

"Nooo, you not! How you feel okay? They chop-a you chest!"

"Uh, thanks very much, Guillermina, I'll talk to you really soon." She means well, she really does. Maybe it's just a language problem.

So there I was: home six days after surgery, bruised in body and spirit, but all the more determined to reconstruct the breast and get on with life. I soon discovered that life in the sheltered hospital environment had indeed kept me in an emotional cocoon. Going home meant being in all those familiar places where I had previously been whole.

Before I left, I had a talk with my surgeon. "Arthur needs to talk to you," I said. "He's feeling fragile. Not at all like a doctor but more like a worried husband." His eyebrows went up. "Well, he should feel wonderful about himself. He found the lump." I knew that, of course, but Arthur needed some "stroking," too. Once I was home, to be able to reach out in the middle of the night and find him on the other pillow was wonderfully comforting. Sex, however, was the furthest thing from my mind. I was still hurting and raw, physically and psychologically.

Without the option of reconstructive surgery, I would have been in much worse shape, psychologically. It still didn't erase this sudden, terrifying glimpse into my own mortality: the realization that, after all the struggling to achieve some measure of immortality, I wasn't going to beat death any more than anyone else, and that I might even die much sooner than I'd planned . . . in mid-flight. I used to say, cavalierly, that when I died I wanted it to be in mid-project, involved in some marvelously stimulating pursuit. What I hadn't realized then was that I would never feel that the current project/flight should be the last. Dying was always going to be too soon. At the same time I experienced sporadic bursts of euphoria—the exultation of just having survived something as dreadful as mastectomy. The anticipation had been so much more terrible than any experience could possibly have been that even death couldn't appear that frightening anymore. I felt a sense of relaxation. I wasn't in great shape, but I was alive and I felt strong in that knowledge. The scar seemed a badge of courage. Those days I thought often of a quote attributed to Mike Nichols: "Life is terrible but interesting."

My favorite *New Yorker* magazine cartoon that week was of a little man in bed at dawn, quilt pulled up to his chin. He looked terrified, and as a group of demons and hobgoblins was flying out the window, one of them waved, calling, "'Bye now, and thanks for thinking of us."

Even before I felt strong enough, I began to work again. I was reminded of that old joke about the patient who asked the doctor if he'd be able to play the piano after surgery. The doctor, surprised, asked if he had played it before, and the patient replied that he hadn't. I guess I had to see if I could still play my "piano" without a breast. The auditions went well and the response was positive. What was my fear? That they would faint when I walked into the room because I'd have "cancer" written in scarlet letters on my forehead? But of course they didn't. I just had to go through the paces and prove that my ability hadn't been altered by the experience, that there was part of me I could still count on.

Historically, when a crisis occurs, I retreat into a fog of manic activity. Then, when my psyche decides that I can handle the situation without being institutionalized, I finally begin to deal with the hard realities. My ex-husband called: "Well, has it come up and hit you between the eyes yet?" I had a vivid mental image of a flying breast aimed at the bridge of my nose. He reminded me that his mastectomy was performed twelve years to the day before I had mine. A numerologist would have a field day with that one! He was actually very supportive and reassured me that he'd be available if I needed moral support. One less supportive acquaintance, a woman, offered, "Don't talk to me about *Cancer!* If I knew you had that, I wouldn't have come to see you. I thought you had a hysterectomy!" I cried that night because remarks like hers touched off all of my dormant hysteria. I knew what it would take to snap me out of my fog and into reality. It would be my first encounter with insensitivity, with people too fragile themselves to be able to shelter me within a warm cocoon of love. I had no margin of flexibility, no elasticity. Arthur patted my left knee and then my right knee in lieu of patting something that might hurt. Actually, nothing hurt, physically. It was more like a bad charley horse, like a pitcher's badly strained arm.

Two weeks after leaving the hospital, I announced to the doctor that, at least physically, I felt like my old self, and if I didn't look down and see something missing, I'd think it had all been a bad dream. Arthur and I were in his office after my examination. Dr. H. sat at his desk across from me. "Well, honey," he said gently, "the pathology people found a little involvement in the lymph nodes. It's minimal, but I think it would be wise to do some chemotherapy." While he was speaking, I watched his lips move, but I felt as though the words were bouncing off a steel plate in my head. I kept thinking that he must have been talking to someone behind me.

He told me that the consensus was that the malignancy had been surgically removed, but since two cancer cells had been detected in one of seventeen examined nodes (thirty-four had been removed), a year of adjuvant chemotherapy was prescribed—just to make sure there weren't one or two little devils lurking somewhere else in my body. He reassured me that I was in the best possible category for survival and that I probably wouldn't lose my thick hair. He also predicted that I would have a premature, drug-induced menopause, since the drugs suppress the multiplication of cells. Hence, no more egg laying. I would probably feel "icky," as he put it, the day after each treatment.

As he spoke, all I could envision was friends standing next to my coffin at my memorial service. I could hear them relating loving anecdotes about me. As I left Dr. H.'s office, I heard myself splutter to him and Arthur that I would be awfully angry if I died.

Those next few weeks, the crying would always start without warning: in the middle of a word, when I'd be talking about something totally unrelated to the cancer. It was like turning on a faucet. I found that I wanted nothing so much as to stay in my room and my bed. That was a new feeling; I'd always wanted to get out and conquer the world. Home had been just a place to change my clothes and get a brief respite before setting out on a new daily campaign. But suddenly home was where I wanted to be all the time and going out was hardest. I would lie there and cry, just thinking how lucky others were not to be crying all the time. I also had a strange new reaction to all of the plants and flowers I received. I wanted to shout, "For God's sake, I'm having enough trouble taking care of me, don't send me another life to be responsible for!"

I couldn't understand why I had a spread of cancer to the nodes when the malignancy had been discovered even earlier than my mother's, and she'd had no lymphatic involvement. I also learned that, even though we'd both had the same type of cancer, I also had a condition called lobular neoplasia, in which all breast tissue is potentially cancerous. This meant my remaining breast was at great risk. I had an image of myself spending the rest of my life palpating my left breast and neck and visiting a specialist every four months just to make sure I didn't grow another cancer there, and then, if I did, hoping that we'd caught it before it spread to the nodes. Dr. H. told me that the current practice was to advocate preventive surgery in cases like mine. However, he added that not many women were able to do that yet. Even from within my fog, I heard myself say, "If I have any chance of cancer showing up in the other breast, I want it to come off." His advice was not to consider that move while on chemotherapy. He explained that the drugs temporarily affect the immune system; resistance to infection is lowered, making surgery a poor risk. Since there had never been a case reported in which a malignancy developed during chemotherapy, he urged me to finish that course before dealing with any more decisions about preventive mastectomy or reconstruction.

Easy for him to say. I couldn't stop thinking about it. I had to plan out my life, as I always do. It infuriated me that I had a different cancer from my mother's. If the tendency toward the disease was familial, then why wasn't it the same kind? Also, when her cancer was discovered she was sixty-five. I was forty-three! I learned that the trend is for the disease to show up about ten years earlier in successive generations. As Arthur would say, medicine is an art rather than an exact science. The current state of the art was all we had to go by. I just had to accept that. I felt like a living example of Murphy's Law during those first few weeks; everything that could go wrong did. I could only view it as a string of betrayals. First, the "harmless cyst" was a malignancy. Second, the "clean" nodes had been slightly sullied by cancer. Third, I had a high risk of disease in the other breast. I even began to have paranoid fantasies about my little group of doctors: the surgeon, the gynecologist, even Arthur. I imagined that they all knew I was a hopeless case and had undoubtedly conspired to keep the truth from me.

I noticed that I felt best when I was at work and in social contact. At those times I was almost euphoric, energetic, and productive. Perhaps I was seeking to confirm my own existence, making sure that I was still the same person to others. Also, when I was with others, I didn't have time to be alone with my own thoughts. During the day I maintained a busy schedule at work, but at night my dreams revealed my worst fears. One stands out in my memory: I was watching a very large, faceless being in monk's robes who sat cross-legged on the floor. In its arms it held a tiny spider monkey, who looked up at it with trust and adoration. Suddenly the robed figure drew a huge pin out of its clothing and began pricking the monkey all over its body. I watched it slowly bleed to death, and as it was dying, it looked up as if to say, "Why are you doing this, what did I do?" When I woke, I remembered that one of the first things Dr. H. told my mother and me, years ago, was that most of his experimental work in breast cancer was done with monkeys.

Before starting chemotherapy, I underwent a bone scan to make sure there were no other areas of malignancy in my body. My first reaction to the test was to associate it with terminal cases only. I had been on such a "bad-news roll" that I couldn't remember what it felt like to hear good news. As I took a seat in the hospital's nuclear medicine department, I noticed there was only one other person waiting. It was a woman dressed in what could only be described as death-defying colors: hot pink, bright green, and dazzling white. A matching scarf covered a head made bald by chemotherapy. She was in her mid- to late forties, pretty, and rather robust. "Bursting with health," I thought. As I sat down, I smiled at her. She leaned toward me and whispered, confidentially, "They don't find out anything good here." Recovering from that rather stunning opener, I said, in my best "Nightingale" manner, "Well, I guess you have to believe that they're trying to find out how to help you." She ignored that, asking, "Are you having a bone scan?" When I acknowledged that I was and told her I'd had a mastectomy, she said, "Oh, I started with that, too. Now they've found spots all over my body. But I waited with that lump for a year and a half before I went to the doctor. Now I know it's everywhere because my bones ache all over." Just then the nurse called my name. As I sat on the examining table, the first question the doctor asked was whether my bones ached anywhere. Thinking of that devastating encounter, I breathed a sigh of relief as I quickly replied, "No, not at all."

Thankfully, my bone scan proved negative, and less than one month after the mastectomy I began a year-long course of chemotherapy. It was to be administered in twenty-eight-day cycles by an oncologist, a physician specializing in chemotherapy. He was a gentle, thoughtful man with a quiet sense of humor. Arthur accompanied me to my first treatment, and the three of us discussed the drug program and potential side effects. The medications all had ominous-sounding names: Fluorouracil, Methotrexate, and Cytoxan. On day one of each cycle, I would receive an intravenous injection of Fluorouracil and Methotrexate, as well as beginning an oral dose of Cytoxan from day one through day fourteen. On day eight, I would return for a second intravenous dose. On day fifteen, I would stop all medication for the next two weeks. The doctor cautioned that women over thirty-five did not usually resume menstruation following chemotherapy. The purpose of the drugs is to suppress the multiplication of cancer cells, but in doing so, other functions depending on cell multiplication cease as well, such as ovulation. Until science determines how to separate these drug reactions, chemotherapy will produce the bad with the good. My periods were another symbol of my youth, my option to bear another child. I bitterly resented this sudden chemical interference. It was difficult to remember that this was a life-saving measure being done *for* me rather than *to* me. I felt as if I had walked out of one room in which I was a young woman full of confidence and optimism, and when I entered the next room, I was old and fearful. What had happened to all those "rooms" in the middle of my life?

My doctor/support system continued to stress the point that every bit of cancer seemed to have been surgically excised from my body. The pathology study was a particularly meticulous and lengthy one. It was unlikely that those two cancer cells in the nodes would have been detected in the more abbreviated studies conducted in most other hospitals. Many doctors believe now that the body's own immune system can successfully conquer those microscopic findings, but knowing those cancer cells were there, I could not ignore them. As I left the oncologist's office after my first treatment, I made a conscious determination to force myself to concentrate on the positives wherever possible. It didn't help much to calculate one visit down, only twenty-three to go. . . . My little family was concerned but supportive regarding the chemotherapy. The children's bickering was considerably reduced and they tried to be helpful at home.

One night Nancy had a particularly vivid anxiety dream. In it we had a special subscription to *The New York Times;* but a *Times* that predicted the events of the following day. Her job was to read the obituaries and tell me whether or not I would die the next day. I decided to take her to visit my doctor so that she could hear, first hand, of the statistics in my favor. Just talking about it seemed to relieve her anxiety. It was particularly difficult for her to deal with the concept of familial predisposition to the disease. My gynecologist was especially helpful. "Look," he told her, "every family has a little black cloud hovering over it. In mine it's heart disease. In yours it's cancer. It's unfortunate that you have to be aware of it this early, but it's just something to be watchful about and to tuck away in a corner of your mind. For you it's nothing to worry about at this point in time. When you're much older, it will be the job of a trained professional. The responsibility will be on his shoulders."

In the beginning I did not confide in friends about the chemotherapy program. Difficult as it was for me to be private, I was fearful that I would be "written off" by friends and potential employers as terminally ill. However, once I became accustomed to the idea and saw that it was not always synonymous with death, I could begin to be more open about it. I have always believed there is nothing in the human condition to be ashamed of, but I, too, had been a victim of cancer's negative public relations. I began to see how secrecy only perpetuates the mystery and ignorance connected with cancer and how I could help provide a positive example of survival and honesty in terms of the disease. Hard times are bad enough without isolating those enduring them. Sharing experiences can only help make them feel less lost. Besides, it was difficult enough to maintain my own equilibrium during this process without the added obstacle of a network of lies. That would have taken much more emotional energy than I could spare.

Chemotherapy dragged on. The predicted cessation of menstruation occurred after three months of treatment and included all of the classic symptoms of menopause. I experienced such an intense inner heat that I was convinced I had a Bunsen burner located right in my middle. All too often an invisible hand would sneak in and turn up the flame when I'd least expect it, bathing me in perspiration. During the two weeks on medication I would feel nauseated, fatigued, and depressed. Once I was off the drugs, those symptoms would gradually subside, and during the day or two preceding the next cycle I would feel marvelous, full of energy and enthusiasm. I could then remember what I used to feel like, the way, I hoped, I would feel when the treatments were all over. No matter how miserable I had been during my two weeks "on," when I felt well again I couldn't recall that sick feeling. Just like childbirth: you remember only the good things. Thank God for selective memory, may it never fail me. I learned to cram as much activity as possible into those two-week respites. During that whole long year, the thought of eventual reconstruction gave me a much-needed focus and a sense of control.

Eric graduated that June from high school. It was less than one month after my surgery, and not surprisingly I was more sentimental than usual. Naomi, my friend and the mother of Eric's classmate, pressed a tissue-wrapped brooch into my palm and closed my fingers over it. It was a hand-painted wooden bird in flight, and the note read: "Maggie dear, you will fly again." How does anyone make it through without friends?

Two and a half months later, Eric left for college. It was a particularly awkward time at which to grapple with the concept of the emptying nest. I told him that even though it was a more complex leave-taking time than we had anticipated, he mustn't feel any reluctance or guilt about going. Just talking about it made it easier for both of us to make the transition. Besides, now it was his time to fly.

Six months into chemotherapy, on Halloween, I detected a lump in my left breast . . . my favorite breast . . . my *only* breast. I was in bed next to a sleeping Arthur and watching one of my all-time favorite films, *Blithe Spirit*, with Margaret Rutherford. I was lying there after having dispensed the last of the Halloween candy to our building's share of witches and goblins. Halloween had been one of my favorite childhood holidays, but I felt so ancient lately that it was difficult to believe that I actually ever was a child! But then I had pictures to prove it. I lay there smiling at the television screen. My arms were crossed over my chest, my fingers resting lightly on the outer side of my last remaining breast. There it was: another hard little lump. "I've got to be imagining this," I thought. "This is a very bad replay!" My next thought was that I was being punished for preferring this breast to the other one in the first place. I woke Arthur, took his hand, and somehow managed to say calmly, "Feel this." He agreed; he could feel the lump. I'd spent a good part of the previous six months relying on the talents of Miss Rutherford, Mel Brooks, and Mike Nichols and Elaine May to make me laugh, but, as I felt that lump, even Miss R. couldn't work her customary magic. Inexplicably, we both fell asleep immediately. There was nothing to discuss; it was too terrible to acknowledge.

The next morning I awoke to feel Arthur stroking my cheek. "You know," he said, "he's going to want to do a biopsy of this." As we drove up to Dr. H.'s office, I kept remembering him saying, "We have yet to hear of a malignancy developing during chemotherapy." After he examined me, he repeated that comforting statement, but he also cautioned that I could be the one exception. Therefore, it had to come out.

I thought only a moment before I said, "Listen, if I have the lump out now, I'm only going to come back in six months to take the whole breast off. I can't deal with this lobular neoplasia factor. I don't see the point of undergoing two procedures with general anesthesia. Each time I think I see an end to this nightmare, something else happens to prolong it. So if we're planning to take the breast off eventually, for God's sake do it now. Even if the lump is benign, just take the whole goddamned thing off. It's become ugly to me, it only reminds me of disease and death." After I'd finished my outburst, he said, quietly, "You've made a very wise decision," but I didn't feel wise, I just felt desperate—and competitive. I felt as if I had to beat this enemy in the biggest contest of my life, and I intended to be the victor. The option of reconstruction gave me the invaluable strength to take that life-saving preventive measure. I knew that I had to do everything possible to rid my body of the specter of cancer before I could get on with my life. I decided that if I were rebuilding one breast, I might as well rebuild two and have them match. They never did before. I chose to see that as a "plus"; I could improve on what I was given in the first place.

Waiting for the surgery, I wanted more than anything else to run away. Every other time in my life I had been able to physically remove myself from a problem: school, work, relationships. But in this instance I had a terrible sense of suffocation, of being constantly surrounded by the threat of disease. I became obsessed with travel ads, brochures describing exotic, faraway places. One day, as I ran to make a subway, I saw an elderly, white-haired gentleman drop his token under the turnstile. I retrieved it for him and he thanked me as we both dashed into the same car. He had a Scandinavian accent and a very kind smile. I asked him where he was from and he replied, "Copenhagen." "Tell me what it's like there," I asked, silently scolding myself for picking up a perfect stranger on, of all places, the subway. He began to describe Tivoli Gardens, as if he knew, by the way I asked, what I needed. It was the most magical description; I could picture it so clearly that I almost believed I had been there myself. We reached my destination, and as I left the train, bidding my friend goodbye, I realized with a sinking feeling that, for the first time in my life, wherever I went, I would take my problem with me. The only respite was my fantasy life.

However, not all of those fantasies were fun. Some nights I lay in bed and had funeral fantasies. Traditionally, I had always believed in cremation after donating everything that still "worked" to cancer research. However, I balked at my organs being used for research purposes only where they might be dissected, hemmed and hawed over, and then discarded. I needed more of a sense of continuity than that! So I'd decided to specify my donations for implantation. In my bid for immortality, it seemed appealing that parts of me could continue life in someone else's body. In my postmastectomy fantasies, however, the cancer society would reject my parts since I'd had the disease myself. "Oh no, my dear," they'd say, "we certainly can't use that body now!" Perhaps, I reasoned, they might still welcome my eyes. My sister, Linda, pointed out that I should send my contact lenses along as well, whereas I thought that the recipient wouldn't notice the myopia, being so thrilled just to see again. Linda's response was "Oh, you know, after the first few days, they'll want to know why they can't read the fine print." My nagging fear is that, if I give away my eyes, I'll probably end up somewhere where I'll need them and I'll have to rely on the guy next to me to tell me what's going on!

My fantasies kept pace with my mounting hysteria. The organ-donation scenario was extended to the cremation fantasy. I speculated that, if my body was accepted, after all, it would leave very little to cremate: perhaps only a couple of toes and an ankle bone, requiring a very small jar for the ashes. What happens then? Does Arthur keep it on his desk as a paperweight? Or on his bedside table, as my childhood neighbor, Mrs. Baker, did? When my mother would take me there for tea, I would wander into the bedroom and stand, absolutely transfixed, by the jar containing the late Dr. Baker. I had the feeling that, if I removed the cover, his round little face with the metal-framed eyeglasses would be smiling up at me. Of course, I could be scattered somewhere. But where? Are they going to want my ashes lying around all over the seats of a Broadway theater? And ever since I got caught in an undertow, I'm petrified of the ocean. Exhausted by my runaway imaginings, I would finally fall asleep, leaving it to someone else to work out.

The night before the surgery I was panicked by the realization that I would never see either of my own breasts again. A breast isn't the sort of item one takes home in a jar. The surgeon suggested that we photograph the breast to provide a model for reconstruction. When one breast is reconstructed, the remaining one is, of course, a model for size and position. However, I was about to lose my model. So, in my hospital room, Arthur used our Polaroid camera to photograph my breast from every possible angle. I slipped that bizarre collection of photos into an envelope labeled "ME; BEFORE," and tucked them away for future reference. A headless, unibreasted me. I had heard that, in some cases, the nipple of the breast being removed could be saved and "banked" for use in eventual reconstruction, when it would be used on the implant or halved in the case of bilateral implants. It seemed ideal until I read an article in one of Arthur's medical journals stating that, occasionally, in a breast prone to disease, the nipple is also at risk. A fantasy ensued in which we saved the nipple and put it on my two new breasts, a cancer then developed in the nipple, and all had been for naught. I discarded the idea immediately. If we were making new breasts, we could make new nipples as well.

After the surgery, a simple mastectomy (removal of the breast only), the surgeon said, "Just think, now you'll never have to worry about breast cancer again." Of course, I no longer had any breasts either, but that seemed far less important. The worry of disease recurrence must have been with me constantly because, even though the lump was benign, I felt relieved to be rid of that breast/time bomb. I told Arthur that, though it was an inappropriate metaphor, I never realized how much that breast had been hanging over my head. When I heard that the growth was benign, I had a momentary twinge of "My God, it didn't have to come off after all, at least not yet," but I still found it preferable to have taken that action than to wait for the cancer to show up again.

The physical recovery from the second mastectomy was much easier than I'd anticipated, and I immediately resumed work. Activity was the best revenge for self-pity. After all, I told myself, except for the removal of the lymph nodes in the first surgical procedure, it wasn't really invasive surgery. Breasts suddenly seemed terribly expendable: just a neat slice off the outside of the body. I spent a good deal of time telling myself that two mastectomies really didn't matter as long as I was disease-free, and intellectually I believed it. There was relief that, having had an excellent surgeon, I was not severely disfigured. Just a perfectly flat, childlike chest with a pink, pencil-thin, horizontal scar on each side. I was still, however, finding it increasingly difficult to adjust to the ever-changing topography of my body: first one breast gone, then the other. In six months my whole image had been altered, and I couldn't keep up with it, even running as fast as I could.

At least everything matched again. After the first mastectomy I had been fitted with a breast prosthesis, but I couldn't bring myself to buy a second one. Instead I just stopped wearing the one I had and accepted a temporary Audrey Hepburn profile. Another prosthesis seemed too final a commitment to being breastless. After the first surgery one of my actor friends had attempted to comfort me with "Well, Mag, you must still have one real cute little one left." No word from him after this procedure! Then there was Gordon, who offered, "Well, you still have great legs." My family was as relieved as I to get it all over with. There is nothing quite as special as my memory of waking and seeing the loving faces of my children, a street vendor's flowers in hand, my sister, and Arthur: my blessed little support group.

I went right back to chemotherapy, didn't even skip a beat. The surgery fell right in the middle of my two weeks off the medication. I had hoped for a little more time away from my "poison," but in the long run I knew that it was better to end the year on schedule than to prolong it. I had exactly six months left. Once I resumed my visits to the oncologist, I found less differentiation between the periods on and off the medication. He explained that there is a gradual buildup of the toxicity level in the system, which reduces the contrast. The fatigue level was constant from then on. I began to anticipate the post-injection nausea before I even reached the office. It was impossible to tell how much of that nausea was real and how much was psychological. I felt like Pavlov's dog with my conditioned reflex.

None of the patients in the oncologist's waiting room were particularly communicative. Of course, that was understandable, since it was no one's favorite place to be. We would all sit there quietly, leafing through magazines, trying to pretend that we were only at the dentist's. Then one of the staff would call out from the back office, "MRS. SNYYYYDER," and I would yell back, "COMMMMING." It reminded me of being called in for dinner when I was a child: sort of comforting.

At times, lying on the examining table, staring up at the same prints on the same wall, it took all the strength I had to stay there and wait for the injection. A little voice inside me would urge, "Quick, he's not here yet. Run!" But then I would force myself to remember that this was being done to help me. Three or four reminders would get me through the visit. I read all of the books telling me that the cancer cell is weak, confused, and wandering and that the chemotherapy would seek it out and destroy it. My kindly oncologist labeled me a "real trooper." As I left, I'd mentally cross one more treatment off my calendar and start for home, a tiny Band-Aid on the needle mark in the crook of my left elbow.

Hanging on to the bus strap one day, I was standing in front of some teenagers on their way home from school. They were staring at the Band-Aid, and it occurred to me that I might be taken for a well-dressed junkie, especially since the Methotrexate darkens the veins on that arm, leaving "tracks." Of course, I had in fact just gotten my "fix." The main difference was that I was about to feel lower instead of higher. I learned how best to deal with the post-treatment nausea, by scheduling my injection for late in the day. The most severe aftereffects set in four to five hours later, and by that time the productive part of my day was over. I would take two to three Compazine tablets to combat the nausea, and sleep through the night. By the next morning the worst of the queasiness had passed, but I still had the feeling that a sixteen-ton weight had been lowered onto my head. It was such a vivid manifestation of the drugs' physical depressants. I had expected the nausea, the chronic fatigue, and even the mouth sores. I could do something to control all of those factors: timing the treatments, limiting my schedule so that I could rest more, and medically treating the sores. I was fortunate in that I did not lose any of my hair and was told that, on this three-drug regime, hair loss was only negligible. I wasn't prepared, however, for the more amorphous side effects; the chemically induced depression and loss of libido. I knew that my hormones would go haywire, but I guess I didn't want to face the consequences of those changes. It might have been easier to bear if I had known that those factors were part of the whole picture for other women in the same situation. But I thought it was just me; I kept trying to talk myself out of it.

One day, after a treatment, I was lying on my bed, utterly miserable and forlorn, when I heard a crash in the living room. I ran in to find that the cats had knocked a photograph of me to the floor. It was in a delicate hand-painted china frame, a birthday gift from my sister. It lay on the floor, face up, with the glass shattered like a jigsaw puzzle over my face. It seemed so prophetic that I just stood over it, sobbing. I felt so fragile myself that I couldn't imagine being able to put the pieces of my life back together again. I felt dried up, mentally and physically, and I worried that those lovely sexual urges would never return. I felt so enervated by the surgery and the chemotherapy that sex just never occurred to me, although I found it both satisfying and enjoyable when I did participate. Arthur was eternally patient and comforting. He reassured me that it would all return with the cessation of chemotherapy and the belief, in time, that I had put the disease behind me. He'd explain, "You've got to believe that you'll live again before you believe in sex again." Arthur has a much healthier sense of perspective than I. Actually, his perspective spans about two thousand years, whereas mine covers the next twenty minutes or so. We strike a nice balance. Throughout the entire experience he never made me feel that my sexuality depended in any way on my breasts. Actually, I have never heard him refer to a woman in purely physical terms but rather in terms of personality, intellect, and character. I know that my illness was a terrible time for him in many ways. Aside from the worry of losing me, he had to put up with my erratic mood shifts. I must have been terrible to live with; for *me* to live with me was a chore. How must it have been for everyone else? Talking about Arthur, I would complain jokingly to friends that living with a saint can be a great burden— one that I've gladly learned to bear, however.

One evening we joined dear friends, a couple, for dinner. The man was being treated for another, more widespread form of cancer than mine and we shared the same oncologist. Because of the toxic effects of the drugs, the doctor's credo was "Six to eight glasses of water a day helps keep kidney damage away." We sat there drinking glass after glass. The busboy must have taken us for refugees from the Sahara.

Many times during the remaining months of chemotherapy, I had to fight the daily impulse to curl up in bed, covers over my head, and just stay there until the nightmare of treatment was over. I always stopped just short of giving in. I forced myself to do everything possible to counteract the negative aspects of treatment. For one thing, I discovered that while I was working I could forget about myself completely. I was extremely fortunate that year in that I worked fairly steadily. No matter how ill I felt in my dressing room before a performance, the moment I walked onstage "in character," I was symptom-free for the duration of the play; like Alice through the Looking-Glass, stepping out of one world and into another. It was the one sure way to get a vacation from myself. During that period I lived by a quote of Twyla Tharp's: "Art is the only way to run away without leaving home." At home I treated myself to the best mattress I could buy on the grounds that, if I was going to spend 90 percent of my time there in bed, then it might as well be in great comfort. I also ate what and when I liked, consistent with the concept of "pleasuring" myself as much as possible. Food was still one of the few sure ways of making myself feel better, and I made a pledge of moderation and exercise when things were back to normal.

It was a struggle to maintain my belief that this treatment was *for* me rather than *to* me when all that I knew, leaving the oncologist's, was that I would become terribly ill about five hours later. It was a difficult concept to grasp in a positive way. I would remind myself that I was fortunate compared to others on more lethal forms of chemotherapy; my reactions were mild compared to theirs. Although as my friend Robbe reminded me, "Just because your back isn't broken doesn't mean your hangnail doesn't hurt."

At times I wondered what the long-range effects of chemotherapy would be. No one can answer that question yet. But what was my choice? My priority at that point was to eradicate the disease. I would deal with the rest later. My doctors continued to reassure me with the statistics for the high cure rate of breast cancer. Women who had an early detection of disease, mastectomy, minimal nodular involvement, and a year of chemotherapy had a 93 percent survival rate based on a five-year follow-up by Dr. Gianni Bonadonna, the Milan physician who developed the progam. My first reaction to that was to ask what would happen after five years. But they'd only been using this drug program since 1976. The difficult concept to grasp is that we have to wait to see how much longer it's successful. I'll be satisfied only when I meet the woman who's lived forty or fifty years after having two breasts removed, two cancer cells in one node out of seventeen, and a year of adjuvant chemotherapy—another me, that is, but many years later. Of course, she doesn't exist. But if I get through the next thirty years or so, they'll have me and a great many others as examples. By then, I hope, they'll have found a cure for cancer.

With many acquaintances, less informed about statistical successes, I had the sense that I was being regarded cautiously, placed "on hold," put on the back burner. I fantasized their thoughts: "Oh, she's okay for a while, but it's probably going to come back, it always does, you know, two operations, chemotherapy, etc." I kept thinking that I had to prove to myself and everyone else that I was going to live; it was exhausting.

At one point I realized that I was extremely competitive with my disease. I had always responded to life's difficulties in that manner: a stubborn, obsessive drive to win out against all odds. If I were to describe my cancer visually, it would be as a faceless competitor in the opposite corner of a boxing ring, gloved fists raised in a fighting posture. The bout was always enervating, but I never stopped believing in my ability to survive.

Paradoxically, the first time I stopped feeling like a cancer victim was with the second mastectomy. I had started taking responsibility for the prevention of the disease by making the final decision to operate. Although surgery was an advised procedure and would not have been done without a valid reason, I could have insisted on holding on to that breast. But I made the decision to finish the course of treatment, to get on with my life, part of which was to end the risk with preventive surgery. I exercised an element of control, and from that moment I negated a good deal of the rage I felt about having cancer. I was in charge, and with that came a satisfying new feeling of strength. Reconstruction seemed to me another step in regaining my pre-cancer confidence and life-style, an effective method of eradicating a negative memory.

3

The Road to Reconstruction

All during that interminable year of mastectomies and chemotherapy I clung to the thought of eventual reconstruction the way I would to a life preserver. Many days when I felt as if I were struggling to keep from "drowning," some early words of my surgeon kept echoing in my memory: "You are an excellent candidate for reconstruction." That promised land just seemed like a very long swim away, but it gave me a much needed direction, a goal to aim for. The advice of both my oncologist and my surgeon was to postpone reconstruction until chemotherapy was over and my immune system had returned to normal. All our efforts were focused on curing the disease during that year, but that didn't keep me from daydreaming about eventual reconstruction. It represented a fitting reward for all that had gone before. However, so much of my energy went into surviving that year that I shelved my reconstruction research until it was almost over. As long as I knew it was mine for the asking, I could afford to wait for the practical details.

In the meantime, during the last few months of chemotherapy, I had ample time to examine my reactions to the whirlwind events of the past year. There was definitely no shortage of anger. It burst forth at unexpected moments, like huge belches. I was enraged at my body; it was the one thing I thought I knew best and it had become a total stranger. My self-image had suffered greatly. I would stare into the mirror, applying makeup mechanically, but if asked to describe the face looking back at me, I would say that I saw absolutely nothing. I looked right through it. Except for one feature: I saw deep hollows underneath my eyes that I had not noticed before. Now all I could visualize was my own skull beneath the skin.

During that time I finally came to realize that I'd been expending a great deal of energy denying the fact that cancer was bound to make a difference in my life. In reality, it had become all-consuming, affecting 100 percent of my existence. I couldn't possibly pretend any longer that it wasn't my primary focus. The pressure of pretending it didn't matter was exhausting. In recognizing that fact, I gave myself permission to ease up, my "You don't have to be Übermensch" lecture. I made an appointment to see a therapist who had helped guide me through previous life crises. I desperately needed help in sorting out my feelings and dealing with my sense of physical and mental vulnerability.

The first question my therapist asked after hearing my nonstop recitation of the year's events was why I had not come to see him sooner. I replied that I could not bear the thought of one more doctor's appointment in my schedule. There were the oncologist, the gynecologist, and the breast surgeon. But I soon realized that my answer was merely an avoidance of the real issue. I had told myself I didn't need therapy, since I openly and often discussed the problem with my friends and family. That was true to a certain extent, but in therapy I knew I would have to deal with all of the terrible anger and fear I was repressing. By myself, I could deal with it only in short bursts. My fear during chemotherapy was that, if I began to let out my rage, I would fall apart. Just living through it was so debilitating, I was afraid that if I let down I wouldn't make it back there for the next month, the next injection. But then, thanks to the subconscious mind, I found myself dialing the psychiatrist's number. I had finally acknowledged that I didn't have to fight the battle all by myself. His perception, sensitivity, and humor proved invaluable. Therapy had always seemed like mental housecleaning to me: picking up a corner of my psychic "carpet" and, one by one, sweeping out piles of dust and debris, smoothing out the rug, lump by lump. Well, at that point there were two fewer lumps on my body but several more under the rug. The therapy helped enormously to illuminate my feelings about my breasts and how I was affected by their loss.

As a young girl, I remember being very self-conscious about my small breasts. In junior high school, when everyone else began to develop breasts, I didn't. I was taller than they, with a long neck, but definitely flatter. I felt like a giraffe. Some who were kinder, usually men, would refer to me as a gazelle. But to me I just looked like a giraffe, and I was fond of standing hunched over in a vain attempt to look smaller. This only resulted in frequent parental admonitions such as, "For God's sake, stand up straight!" usually delivered in the preteen department of Lord and Taylor's.

There was only one other girl in school with breasts as small as mine. She played the glockenspiel in the marching band. I remembered seeing her one Friday, as flat as ever, and feeling a kind of sad commiseration. But the next day, to my astonishment, she arrived at the football game in a short-sleeved white angora sweater with the biggest, pointiest breasts I'd ever seen. They had grown overnight, as if she'd ingested a new wonder drug. It didn't matter to me that she was wearing "falsies"; I was green with envy. It was small comfort that, when she played the glockenspiel that afternoon, her breasts kept getting in the way. After my mastectomies, all I could think of was what a waste of time that teenage obsession with breast size had been now that I was back to no breasts at all. It's one good reason never to wish for a crystal ball, but giving up my breasts was still preferable to risking my life. Throughout the mastectomy-chemotherapy experience, I reminded myself, over and over, of my basic credo: "Life is my number one priority," and intellectually I never stopped believing it. I kept telling myself that losing my breasts should make no more difference to me than losing a lung or a colon to cancer. As long as I was disease-free, I could resume life pretty much as I had always known it. I kept denying the subversive and widespread implications of being breastless.

I had never considered my breasts to be a particularly critical factor in terms of my achieving sexual satisfaction, and I gratefully discovered after mastectomy that I had an ample number of erogenous zones still in perfect working order. Arthur was a gentle, patient lover, as always, and I had no difficulty achieving sexual satisfaction (a much-needed release during those trying times). Orgasm, a classic amnesiac-of-the-moment, gave me a mini-vacation from my troubled thoughts about mortality. However, I was never the one to initiate lovemaking. Not only was I constantly exhausted from the drugs, but my bygone breasts were a loaded issue during sex—not for him but for me. During that time my body image was that of a large, faceless head placed directly atop two little feet with nothing at all in between. At times that dwarflike figure would appear in my dreams. Nothing about it resembled the "me" I had known. In fact, the head was that of a man but I knew, indisputably, that it was me. I reasoned that the sole purpose of the feet was to provide instant mobility so as to avoid being trampled or trapped. My torso had been mentally displaced. It was too painful a reminder of what had once given me pleasure and was now synonymous with frailty.

This adversely affected my attitude toward sex, even though Arthur continued to be understanding. Foreplay just lost all of its appeal. As a young girl, I thought of foreplay as a man's way of telling me he admired my body and giving himself pleasure. Then I became educated to the fact that, when a man cared for me, foreplay was intended to be mutually pleasurable. I still knew many women who believed that men did not do such things for a woman's enjoyment, only for their own satisfaction. But that had not been part of my thinking for years before mastectomy. However, after surgery, I slipped back to that medieval concept. When foreplay was initiated, I would find myself thinking, "Why is he doing that? It can't be giving him any pleasure. There isn't anything there." I still liked sex but I didn't want to do the fooling around before intercourse. It only served to remind me of what had happened. I considered sex to be a celebration of the body, and at that point I saw nothing to celebrate.

Poor Arthur couldn't win; if he caressed my chest, I'd tell myself that he was just trying to be kind, and if he didn't touch it, I'd assume that he was repulsed by it. I felt like such a nonwoman and hated myself for not being able to intellectualize myself out of that feeling. I think no matter what a loving partner did, it would have been misunderstood. However, talking about it helped us a great deal.

At times, on the way to the shower, I'd catch a glimpse of my naked self in the mirror. I never consciously avoided looking at my chest; it just never stopped being a surprise. It was such a shock that I'd gasp and then cry just because my once pretty body would never be the same again. Like many women, I had always been somewhat critical of my body, but it was mine and it had represented youth and health. Now it had become a constant reminder of my ordeal with cancer, my confrontation with my own mortality. In the very beginning I would forget that I'd lost a breast. I'd wake in the morning with no immediate memory of what had happened. Years ago I'd had a mole removed from the back of my neck. I could never see it, but it had been there since I was born and, even when it was taken off, I still thought of it as being part of me. For a very long time I'd carefully avoid irritating it with my hairbrush as I'd always done. Like my breast, it had been an integral part of my body image. I couldn't even bear losing an earring! How could I accept the loss of a breast?

Simultaneous with the sense of loss, there was tremendous relief that it wasn't a horrible disfiguration but just a flat little chest with a pencil-thin pink horizontal scar. I had a surprising need to reveal it to some of my friends. A few were initially wary, but in every case, when I did reveal it, they expressed astonishment because what they had imagined was far worse. Not only had the act relieved me, but I felt as though I'd performed a service, abolished a myth. In reporting this to my therapist, he described the breast loss as "a massive assault on my sexual integrity." My surgeon termed it a "triple whammy." Not only had I had cancer, he explained, but I was an amputee and a sexual amputee as well. He reminded me that it was the first time I had been hit hard by something I couldn't control; I had been afflicted. I became more aware of other amputees. I'd always felt sympathy for them, but now I felt empathy. I was fortunate; my amputation was not visible. It was as if I'd suddenly become a member of a new club, but one that I'd never cared to join. I thought of Groucho Marx, who announced that he wouldn't join any club that would have him as a member. After the first mastectomy I had begun to count breasts automatically as I walked down the street: two, four, six, eight, and I'd invariably end up with something like seventy-nine. Me, odd woman out. I was enraged at the inequity, literally and conceptually. Giving up the breast voluntarily didn't cancel out the anger associated with the loss. Statistics told me that there were a lot of other seventy-nines out there, but as long as I didn't know all those other women, I couldn't quite believe it.

My sessions with my therapist enabled me to face my feelings of loss in terms of my breasts, and once I had accepted those feelings, I could acknowledge my desire and right to replace them. For me there was more of a feeling of victimization associated with the surgery than with the disease. After all, my life had been saved! Why did I have such trouble holding on to that? I finally concluded that my inability to deal with the victory over disease instead of dwelling on the breast loss was due to my view of my own death as ephemeral and unreal in contrast to the more tangible change in body shape. When my body was altered so drastically, I felt I no longer recognized myself. Reconstructive surgery promised to be the most logical and satisfying means of erasing that constant physical reminder of disease, as well as of soothing an altered ego.

Just before the end of chemotherapy, I made an appointment to discuss my reconstruction with Dr. H. How different I felt, sitting in that sun-washed consulting room discussing such a positive procedure. It helped a great deal to obliterate the painful memory of mastectomy. Dr. H. explained that, not having lost any muscle, I was a candidate for a simple reconstruction procedure, one that involved the insertion of silicone implants in a pocket created behind the pectoral muscle. This could be accomplished in a single procedure and would involve a few days' hospital stay. If I wanted to replace the nipples and areolae, that would be done at a later date after any swelling from the implant insertion had subsided.

I knew that breast surgeons often performed simple implant insertions on women whose mastectomies they had performed. Dr. H. explained, "It gives me such great pleasure to give back what I've had to take away." I felt so thoroughly comfortable and confident with this gentle man who had saved my life that I chose him to do the first stage of my reconstruction, the insertion of the implants. Also, I hadn't the stamina to interview more doctors at that point; I had a bad case of surgeon saturation. At that meeting, Dr. H. showed me photographs of breasts that he had rebuilt. He explained that, in reconstruction, my mastectomy incision would be partially reopened and a flexible silicone sac implant (resembling a jellyfish, I thought) would be inserted. In time the thin scar would fade from deep pink to white and the saline solution filling the implant would exchange freely with my body's cellular fluid. That pleased me, since it made the implant seem less like a foreign object than an active part of me. Dr. H. told me that it was even possible to perform reconstructive surgery on women with radical mastectomies (removal of the breast, lymph nodes, and pectoral muscle) by replacing the lost muscle with a similar one brought from the back (the latissimus dorsi) and then inserting an implant underneath it.

At that time Dr. H. mentioned a newer, more experimental method of reconstruction that utilized a transplanted apron of abdominal fat and blood vessels covering the intestines (the omentum). The aim of this procedure was to re-create a breast mound without the need for an implant, using all natural tissue. It was also used to provide protection over an implant to avoid its being placed behind the pectoral muscle. When I mentioned this to my friends, I was deluged with generous, albeit inappropriate and unfeasible, offers of their unwanted flesh, thighs, hips, and so on. Everybody wanted to change something! At first thought it sounded like an ideal way to achieve a "tummy tuck" and regain my breasts at the same time. However, it involved a much lengthier surgical procedure, with size and symmetry extremely difficult to achieve. There had been reports of the transplanted fat "melting," being reabsorbed by the body, resulting in unpredictable shrinkage of the breast, so together we decided on the more dependable silicone sacs. I was also reluctant to create more scarring, a disadvantage of the omentum reconstruction.

The breasts in the photographs were wonderfully symmetrical and very natural in appearance except for one notable difference: they had no nipples. When I questioned that fact, Dr. H. replied that, since sensation is lost in the mid-breast area after mastectomy, many women are concerned mainly with regaining the fullness and symmetry of the breasts. Also, creating a nipple-areola complex would require a second procedure performed by a plastic surgeon. So re-creating the most natural appearance would entail two stages: (1) the implant insertion and (2) the grafting of skin to create a nipple-areola.

I was tempted to forgo the second procedure, having had it with surgery, but, fearing that with nippleless breasts I would remind myself of the nose of a 747, I decided on a two-stage reconstruction. Two or three months after the insertion of the implants, a plastic surgeon would reconstruct the nipples and areolae. The purpose of the interval was to allow any swelling to subside so that the placement of the nipple could be accurately determined. I had no desire to end up looking like the naked lady in the *New Yorker* cartoon whose gentleman friend, observing that her nipples stared at each other rather than out front, asks if she has consulted an ophthalmologist. Dr. H. told me that he could refer me to a plastic surgeon for the second stage of reconstruction, which would require a few days' hospitalization. (Today, with much progress having been made, the nipple-areola grafts are most often done on an outpatient basis, with the patient returning home in two to three hours, after local anesthesia. Even a simple implant insertion requires only two days in hospital, a great improvement from my time in the "olden days.")

I decided to take one step at a time and wait until after the first stage of reconstruction to meet the plastic surgeon, Dr. S. Dr. H. said that both he and Dr. S. would follow my recovery after the implant insertion, with the latter taking over for the nipple-areola grafts. He emphasized that the aim of reconstruction is to achieve a "match" with the remaining breast. Well, I had a distinct advantage in that case, having nothing left to match. We could create new breasts from ground zero, as it were. I thought, longingly, of reconstruction as an opportunity to fulfill a fantasy. I'd always coveted breasts that were more symmetrical than my natural pair. I never would have elected to do that type of cosmetic surgery before, but now I had the opportunity to create synthetic but super breasts. What a way to get it!

As I left Dr. H.'s office that day, visions of reconstructed "747" breasts dancing in my head, I realized that I hadn't set a date for the reconstruction. I felt that I needed more time— time to recover from the past year before embarking on this new venture.

4

Reconstruction at Last

We selected a date two and a half months after the end of chemotherapy for the reconstruction. That would provide enough time for me to regain a good deal of my former energy. Also, Arthur and I badly needed a second honeymoon, a complete rest and recuperation from the tension of the previous year and a half. The weeks flew by, and as the date for reconstruction drew near, I was both excited and terrified at the prospect. I was feeling stronger and more like the old me each day. The night before the operation, Dr. H. came into my hospital room to discuss the placement of the implants with Arthur and me. This was the time to consult the photographs taken before the second mastectomy. He then drew the plans on my chest with a ballpoint pen and, when we had concluded our discussion, began to wipe the ink off with an alcohol-saturated cotton pad. Watching him, I flinched, feeling a surprising sense of loss. He said, gently, "Well, we can't leave it on there for the operation, can we?" Even though I knew he was making perfect sense, it still felt, for a moment, as if he were taking my breasts away again.

The next day, the surgery went smoothly but, waking up, I discovered that the mastectomies had been painless by comparison. For two days I remained in a medicated fog for what felt like a very severe charley horse, as if several linebackers had been invited to stomp on my chest and back with their boots. To insert the implants, a pocket is created behind the pectoral muscle, necessitating a fair amount of cutting and rearranging in the process. By the third day the discomfort had completely subsided, and I was home five days after surgery. (Today, many women feel able to leave the hospital the day after the reconstruction.) My new breasts were not heavily bandaged, as I'd imagined, but were covered by a thin layer of gauze. Although this had been a somewhat longer procedure than either mastectomy, requiring more anesthesia and causing more discomfort, I recovered in a much shorter time. I was constantly aware that, this time, we were rebuilding, no longer taking away. The most amazing thing was that, from the moment I awoke after the reconstruction, I could no longer remember what it felt like to be without breasts. That made it all worthwhile.

As I recovered, though, two facts became disappointingly apparent. During the next six weeks I developed a good deal of scar tissue around the right implant, causing it to become unnaturally firm and distorted in shape. I thought I could feel it gradually tighten into a hard, fibrotic ball. This, I learned, can occur frequently and unpredictably, unrelated to surgical expertise. (Today measures can be taken to greatly reduce the chances of this happening.) Also, in terms of breast size, I was considerably smaller than before the mastectomies. I was at fault in that I had not made my needs specific enough when discussing size with my surgeon. I had left that decision strictly up to him. There are also several important considerations that help to determine implant size. First, there must be sufficient skin on the chest to cover the implant easily; and second, the sac should not be so large that it will be in danger of extruding from underneath the muscle. If I had not developed the scar tissue, I would probably have settled for my new very tiny breasts. But when it became obvious that the right side would have to be redone when I had the second procedure, I decided to have the plastic surgeon replace both implants with those comparable to my earlier brassiere size, a

B cup. It was disappointing to consider starting over, but since I had already accepted the concept of a two-stage procedure, I felt that, having come so far, I should aim for complete satisfaction.

My sister encouraged me tremendously. My immediate postsurgical reaction was to decide that I couldn't go through it all again, that it was probably just my imagination, they must all look that way. But Linda kept pushing me on. She gave me the courage to redo the implants, as Dr. H. advised. As for Arthur, he couldn't bear the thought of my being disappointed, so he encouraged me to take the necessary steps to remedy the situation. He just wanted me to be happy.

I then had several examination-discussions with Dr. S., the plastic surgeon who was to complete the reconstruction. As planned, he and Dr. H. had both followed my recovery from the first stage and conferred on future treatment. This time I was more outspoken about my needs. His explanations were thorough, and he was always realistic in his descriptions of what I could and could not expect. Since he was grafting the nipples and areolae, he would also replace the implants. As to size, he said that only when he saw the pocket behind the muscle could he tell whether I could accommodate the 300 milliliter size (equivalent to a full B cup). Premastectomy, I had been an asymmetrical 34B. We agreed that he would also keep a 250 milliliter pair of implants ready and use whichever he considered appropriate. The nipples were to be grafted from a microscopic scraping of tissue from the vaginal labia, comparable in texture and color. Dr. S. assured me that, once it was healed, even my gynecologist would be unable to detect any scarring on the vaginal graft site. Waiting the three months after the first reconstructive procedure would ensure accurate placement of the nipple-areola, as well as normal blood circulation in the implant area, facilitating the "taking" of the grafted skin.

The options for the areola graft included skin from the ear lobe or the inner thigh. However, I didn't have enough skin to spare from the ear and the inner-thigh grafts were likely to leave a visible scar. Therefore, Dr. S. suggested the area on the lower right abdomen over the appendix. The resulting pencil-thin scar would not be visible even in a bikini. Over the next few weeks I interviewed several women who had undergone reconstruction, as well as a woman surgeon who had performed hundreds of such operations. I should have done all of that research before the first procedure, but I'm historically lazy that way. I always trusted that things would just work out, that other people would "make it right." I was now finally beginning to assume that responsibility myself.

The surgeon I consulted was affiliated with Memorial Sloan-Kettering Cancer Institute. I had not been back there since I filmed the Xerox commercial. Linda came along for much-needed support. The minute I entered the hospital, all those memories came flooding back. I sat there waiting in the admitting section where we had been shooting and remembered all of the children with one leg or no hair watching us. Unfortunately, the rules required that I had to register as a patient of the hospital even though I was there only for a consultation. That only increased my anxiety, since I felt as if I were going back into the hospital for surgery. I sat there with my ever patient sister and filled out what seemed like a million insurance forms. The only positive aspect was that I was so busy I hardly had a chance to dwell on the other terrified people in the waiting room: women wearing turbans to cover heads rendered hairless by chemotherapy, and new patients with that familiar look of frozen terror. I kept having to fight the thought that I was one of them, repeating to myself over and over, "Yes, I had cancer, but I don't have it *now!*" The surgeon was large, energetic, and very pleasant. She kneaded my breasts like dough and agreed with the plan that my plastic surgeon had outlined. I felt optimistic once more. She also confirmed my feeling that the size I wanted was feasible and appropriate and that, although fibrosis, or capsular contracture, was a frequent complication in such surgery, it need not happen the second time around.

Two months to the day after the first reconstructive procedure, I was back in the hospital for what we all hoped would be the final step. Though Arthur and the children continued to be as loving and supportive as ever, I was anxious to complete this phase of my recuperation so that we could all get on with our lives. In my hospital room the night before surgery, I was filled with so much nervous energy that I pulled the curtains off the three windows, washed them in the bathtub with a tiny bar of Ivory soap, and rehung them. It did wonders for my anxiety, even though I did have a moment or two of doubting my sanity.

The next day I awoke with wonderful breasts (the surgeon had been able to use the 300 milliliter implants), nipples, and areolae all in place; it felt like every birthday gift rolled into one (or two, more accurately). The doctor told me that during the procedure everyone in the operating room voiced their opinion on appropriate implant size and position, viewing me from all sides, arms up, down, and extended. The result was superb! The graft sites were only mildly uncomfortable, the vaginal area feeling as though I had scratched myself with a fingernail. As for the thin scar line over my appendix, the surgeon promised that it would not be visible even in a bikini. For two days I experienced the same back and chest pain as before.

I had wonderful, caring nurses, one of whom, Miss Meade, had cared for my mother after her mastectomy. I promised to return for a visit when the bandages were taken off and the stitches removed. The nurses were just learning about this new form of rehabilitative surgery and were anxious to see the finished product. With their expert care I grew stronger each day. The discomfort from the graft donor sites was only briefly annoying, and after the first couple of days I had no pain in the chest area at all. I just felt fatigue from the general anesthesia and relief that it was finally all over.

Five days later I was home and delighted that I had done the complete procedure. My breasts were healing quickly, firm but not overly so, with no sign of complications. The surgeon instructed me to wear a brassiere during the first few weeks of healing, although, once healed, I would never again need one for support. I had to wonder if, at ninety-five, my breasts would still be firm and uplifted while my rear end had long since dropped to my knees! If so, I could finally qualify then for the *Guinness Book of World Records:* Woman with Longest Torso.

In the weeks that followed, I saw many positive changes in myself. My posture improved dramatically and I moved with more confidence. I was no longer self-conscious when hugging my friends and relatives. I had been painfully aware of my hard, unyielding rib cage pressing up against their bodies. Now there was a lovely maternal cushion there again, and I was surprised to realize how important that aspect of reconstruction was to me, even more important than reestablishing my sexual identity. There was no doubt, though, that I felt more womanly, sexier. I could begin to enjoy admiring glances when I wore the low-cut necklines, strapless dresses, and bikinis that I had assumed I would never wear again. In a new way, my breasts once again became an erogenous zone. Although feeling was still absent in the mid-breast area, my brain could now make the connection between a caress and past sensation. I could recall that sense of pleasure. The nature of my fantasies began to change, too. Instead of being concerned with death and endings, I was thinking of sex and life again. How lovely to welcome back my libido! Looking into the mirror, I began to see my image once more; I was recognizing myself again, permitting myself to be seen. As I walked down the street one day, my hands involuntarily flew up to my chest to make sure my new breasts were still there. For a time after surgery, I would experience moments of panic that they were just a figment of my imagination or that I would wake one day to find that they had vanished. My rational self found it curious that I had so quickly and completely adopted these two silicone-sac breast substitutes as my own. They triggered all of the same irrational responses I had felt for my natural breasts.

While I was breastless, I would often catch a glimpse of

myself in a mirror and see my hand or arm held protectively across my chest. After the reconstruction, my therapist commented on my pre- and postreconstruction body language. Before, he noted, I slouched or curled up in the chair to hide the middle of my body. In contrast, he observed that now I would often put my hands behind my head and stick out my chest. I laughed, embarrassed, never realizing that I had been that obvious. I couldn't deny it, though, because I did feel completely different.

Two incidents that have occurred since my reconstructive surgery illustrate the polarity of reaction to this form of rehabilitation. The first was when I volunteered my services as a speaker at the postmastectomy clinic in my neighborhood YM-YWHA. To my surprise, the man in charge of the physical education program did not appear overly enthusiastic. Instead he said, "You'll probably be interested to know that we have a new curtained area in the ladies' locker room for people like you. Now you can dress and undress without embarrassment." I felt my anger rising as I replied that I saw no reason to hide my body, that having had cancer and plastic surgery was nothing to be ashamed of. He was astonished. "You mean to say that you walk through that locker room in front of those other women? That's terrific!" I congratulated myself on educating him until he added, "Why, I'll bet that every woman who sees you goes right home and calls her doctor for a breast examination!" That was over two years ago, and as I predicted, he has never called me in to speak.

The second incident concerns a beautiful Milwaukee woman I'd met before my cancer was discovered. She was in her mid-forties and had undergone a mastectomy six years earlier. She had adjusted extremely well to the loss, and when I commented on how refreshing it was to meet someone so open about cancer, she said, "Look, I'm fine, I survived the disease, I have a husband who makes me feel wonderful and sexy, and I have a very good life." We laughed together as she recalled her annoyance when, as she shoveled snow away from her car, her prosthesis fell to the ground when she leaned over. She said, "I looked around to see if anyone was watching, picked it up, dusted it off, and stuck it back in. But it's at times like those that it's a damn nuisance!" It was conveniently prophetic because I took great courage from her when, two months later, I learned of my own cancer. Hers was the only truly liberated example I had to follow. We corresponded all through my surgery, chemotherapy, and reconstruction. When I wrote her about my plans for plastic surgery, she replied saying that if she were closer to one of the larger surgical centers, she would have had a reconstruction also. But it meant going away from home, and that was just one more obstacle to overcome.

However, shortly after I wrote her of my successful experience, I received similar news from her. She wrote: "You gave me the courage to go ahead. I found an excellent plastic surgeon in Milwaukee, he rebuilt my breast, and I feel absolutely marvelous! I wouldn't have been able to do it without you." That was one of the most satisfying results of my experience: the knowledge that I might be able to influence other women. I have discovered that most women who have undergone reconstructive surgery are so enthusiastic that they can't wait to discuss it, a sign that it is a tremendously effective form of psychological as well as physical rehabilitation.

One of the most insidious side effects of cancer is the impotent anger felt by the individual. Taking as positive a step as reconstructive surgery helps enormously to alleviate that rage. It cannot negate the experience, but it can certainly create a sense of having more control in an otherwise victimizing situation. It can help to turn negative feelings into positive energy, a critical element in the survival process. I still have anger about having had cancer in the first place, but, without reconstruction, I feel I would have carried the memory of disease around with me much longer than necessary.

Once I recuperated from the surgery (the effects of general anesthesia more than anything else), I began a regime of daily exercise—swimming, running, aerobics. I felt good about my body again, as if I had regained a long-lost friend. Some of my friends were still somewhat cautious, underlining "healthy" on my birthday cards. Most of the time I could no longer remember my glimpse of how close death could be, an image I had so often and so vividly during my course of treatment.

I learned, however, that reconstruction alone is not the key to total tranquillity in terms of cancer. Doubts about recurrence of the disease still persist. The periods of anxiety are of shorter duration, but they still occur. Every so often, when I'm in the shower washing under my arms, I feel what I think is a lump. Each time it turns out to be nothing, but in that instant my death flashes before me again. A second before, I was standing there worrying about whether I'd get a job I wanted badly and all the other things that make up garden-variety paranoia, and suddenly nothing matters again but living. It's certainly one quick way to get your priorities in order. If I read about someone, particularly a woman, dying of cancer, my immediate thought is "Well, her case was different, that won't happen to me." Then a tiny voice whispers, "Are you sure?" and I wonder. Perhaps this is just another case of rationalizing the realities. I have always marveled at how those with terminal disease manage to deny the fact for so long. They hold on to the few statistics supporting their survival as long as they can. I don't really think I am in that category, but a tiny, occasional doubt remains that maybe I am denying also and this will be one big, bad black joke on me.

A surprising aspect of the entire experience was that I waited until reconstruction was finished to finally come to terms with all of the depression associated with having had cancer. I thought that if I let down and let it all out while I was still facing additional treatment and surgery, then I'd have no hope of making it through. After the second phase of reconstruction there was nothing to prevent me from reacting. It was the old familiar feeling of having mistakenly hoped that any desired goal would solve all problems—"If I can just get that job, that divorce, have a child," etc. Then the wish is granted, and as wonderful as it is, it isn't the answer to everything. My goal during treatment and reconstruction was to win out over my adversary and put the experience completely behind me. Having won my battle, I felt oddly empty without that fight for a focus. Also, I was naïve to think that, emotionally, I could ever return to the pre-cancer me. It was impossible to remain unchanged by such a profound experience.

I remember reading *Widow* by Lynn Caine, the book in which she detailed so well the emotional phases through which a widow passes. I realized that those same phases (shock, denial, anger) apply to any loss, whether a relationship, a dream, or even breasts—anytime one is left with a void. Time eventually fills in some of the emptiness. First the pain, then the growth. After all, there have to be some benefits for a painful experience. Somehow we never learn from the good times.

I nursed my post-disease depression for a time until one day, while traveling on a city bus, I pondered the persistent gray cloud still hanging over me. After all, I reasoned, as we lurched up Madison Avenue, I was well again, looking forward to an interesting career and life, more in love with my husband than ever. My family was healthy, my children were doing well. What was it that was still between me and contentment, tugging me back toward depression? Suddenly, standing in that swaying bus, I had a quick glimpse into the center of that cloud. It was divided in two: the first part was my fervent desire never to have had cancer, the wish that it had just never happened. The second element was my yearning to return to the familiar "me," the woman with all of her pre-cancer illusions intact. Well, there was no way I could have either of those wishes granted. I have no power to turn back the clock. But I could see that the wishing had paralyzed me. Having made that realization, it was a liberating feeling to just give myself permission to let it go. If that was the only barrier between me and contentment, then it was also within my control to counteract it. All I had concentrated on were the ways in which I had changed without granting that many of those changes had been positive. To begin with, I had restored my former bust line with reconstruction. I felt that having come through all that I had experienced in those fifteen months proved that I had the strength to get through anything in life. Most of all, by taking a positive, renewing action, I had stopped waiting for someone or something to rescue me. I was finally doing that all by myself! I was emancipated, no longer "at the mercy of."

I realized that, even though I still loved acting, my motivation had changed. I used to act to get away from someone I didn't particularly like: me. Being anyone else was better than being myself. Now that I was beginning to enjoy my own company, there was no need to keep looking for the raison d'être outside myself. A job used to be a matter of life and death, a man the same. No more. Now life-and-death was *really* life-and-death.

All these new feelings were discomfiting only because I had so little in common with the old me. There were no familiar sign posts. I felt the way I used to at every new step, as if I were standing on a diving board over a huge pool without knowing whether there was any water underneath me. But I had to jump. There was no turning back. Life had forced me to the end of that board, and there was no place to go but forward. There wasn't any way I could undo what had happened, so, even though I was terrified of what lay ahead, I had no choice but to go ahead and meet the new me.

Friends corroborated the positive change. One, an engagingly frank director who had known me for years, said, "I don't know if this makes any sense to you, but you look like you're more inside your face." It was a wonderful confirmation of what I already felt: a new sense of my own strength. For me reconstruction was the real and symbolic manifestation of winning out over breast disease, and I had done it! I was no longer reaching frantically outside of myself for strength. Instead, I was providing my own.

I find it curious that taking action in the form of preventive surgery and reconstruction is described by some individuals as a form of bravery. In my case it had merely to do with survival, with getting through as best I could. To my mind it would have been much more difficult to wait for fate to take its turn. I could have sat back and waited to see if cancer developed in the second breast or just continued to feel sorry for myself instead of choosing reconstruction. But then, I'm not long on passivity. I'm often told that I obsess to the distress of others and that I am stubborn to a fault. Ask my family! But I'm beginning to see that that quality is, at least partially, why I'm still here. My father used to say, "You don't know the meaning of the word 'moderation.'" And as a child I considered that a fault. Fault or virtue, it has been my greatest ally. There are two basic styles of dealing with adversity: passive and active. Two ways in which a passive individual might react are depression and denial. Both would avoid confronting the issue at hand. The more active reaction would be to fight the adversity stubbornly, steadily, in the belief that you could ultimately win, the sense that, basically, you deserve good fortune rather than bad. I have found that attitude determines outcome in many instances in my own life.

Taking this theory one step further, does this mean, then, that reaction to adversity is predetermined by one's traditional view of life? In that case, being pessimistic or optimistic by nature would determine the degree of competitive spirit. Mental attitude has been demonstrated to play an important role in healing. Is it then possible for individuals with a traditionally negative attitude to change their outlook by positive example in order to effectively fight disease and make optimistic decisions regarding treatment? I feel blessed in having all my life had an optimistic outlook, believing that I can make anything happen if I try hard enough. Even so, a day did not go by during treatment when I did not think despairingly that I would have liked nothing better than to curl up in bed and sleep for six months. But each time something stopped me from giving in to that urge. I have known other women who, faced with the terror of breast cancer, ran the other way or settled for less treatment than advised. On the other hand, perhaps I did even more than I had to. Who knows? What I do know is that I chose the most comfortable course of action for me, the one my conscience dictated. Life never stopped being the number one priority.

This is not to say that losing my breasts was unimportant. Some feminists argue that a woman doesn't need breasts to be a woman, but it's easy to utter such a statement from a double-breasted position. All I knew was that a part of me was missing and, damn it, I wanted it back! I am also a lousy gambler. I was a poor risk with my particular type of cancer for anything short of bilateral mastectomy. Perhaps others would be able to form the eventual basis for statistical success with less drastic forms of treatment, but I could not be sure that less was not a gamble. Reconstruction, for me, was the satisfying solution to being safe but not sorry.

It is now three years since my reconstructive surgery and over four years since the detection of cancer. I feel wonderful! I find it hard to believe that there was ever a breastless time for me. The scars are barely discernible, the breasts feel natural to the touch, and I have regained a good deal more sensation. Until we have a cure for cancer or sufficient long-term evidence to prove conclusively that other forms of treatment are as effective as mastectomy for eradication of the disease, I can only hope that more women will take advantage of this lifesaving option of reconstruction. Breasts, after all, can be replaced. Lives cannot.

5

Lumpectomy Versus Mastectomy

Breast reconstruction has been such a thoroughly satisfying experience for me on so many levels that, to my mind, my greatest contribution would be to inform as many other women as possible of this option so that each could make her own educated decision. My being so evangelistic does not mean that this will be an appropriate choice for everyone. I realized almost immediately that most women knew too little of this option to even consider it. A 1979 National Cancer Institute survey reported that only 23 percent of all women were even minimally acquainted with the technique of breast reconstruction. If I, knowing that I could rebuild my diseased breast, was paralyzed with fear before surgery, imagine how hopeless and filled with despair the woman is who knows nothing at all of this medical advance. Would it not greatly interfere with her judgment in making the decision on how most thoroughly to ensure herself a disease-free future? If she were educated about reconstruction, would it not be reasonable to expect that she could manage, fearful as she was, to consult a doctor as soon as she became suspicious of breast changes? In that way, breast reconstruction can truly be considered a lifesaving option. At a time when each of us, faced with breast surgery of any kind, feels more emotionally fragile and confused than ever before, I wanted to offer assistance by putting as much information as possible between the covers of one book about the state of the art of reconstruction. Chalk it up to my irrepressible instinct for mothering, undoubtedly borrowed from my own irrepressible mother. The point is that the better informed the patient, the more control she has over the situation, be it breast cancer surgery or breast reconstruction. With knowledge comes less fear of the unknown and the ability to participate more actively in the decision-making process.

I wish now that I had taken the time while waiting those two weeks before my own biopsy-mastectomy to research reconstruction, but I had no such example to follow. Also, there were not as many reconstructive choices available; the technique was still in its infancy. My type of cancer left no choice other than mastectomy as far as I or my doctors were concerned, but at least I could have informed myself about whatever rehabilitative options were available to me. It would have made those two weeks more productive, less fraught with a sense of impotence. At least now, with my experience and that gleaned from those dedicated to helping women return to a pre-cancer life quality, I can attempt to shed some more light on an area that, until now, has been only dimly illuminated.

If every surgeon agreed that there was only one effective way to eradicate breast cancer and rebuild the breast, a discussion of breast reconstruction would be fairly short and simple. However, the field has become increasingly complex, encompassing a whole spectrum of surgical options and reconstructive techniques. The choices for treatment include irradiation (X ray) with or without lumpectomy (tumorectomy), partial mastectomy (quadrantectomy), and mastectomy of varying degrees: simple, modified radical, or Halsted radical. These procedures can also involve chemotherapy in case of positive lymph node findings. Some mastectomies may also require radiation treatment if the cancer has spread to the sternum, or mid-chest, area. All in all, there is quite an alarming array of choices for any woman to consider, but then there are multiple types of breast cancer, each better suited to one form of treatment than another. The choice for breast reconstruction is dependent, in part, upon the method chosen for disease eradication. Therefore, I thought it best to investigate some of the pros and cons offered by experts in the treatment of the cancer. The type of cancer must, of course, be considered when determining the treatment. A woman must know how her particular involvement has traditionally responded to different forms and combinations of surgery/chemotherapy/radiation.

Even though the early lumpectomy-radiation statistics are promising, it has been stated by the most enthusiastic advocates of limited surgery that this procedure is not for everyone. Mastectomy is still the "gold standard" of breast cancer treatment. I was not able to live with the stress of a high-risk situation; I chose the most recommended surgical course for me since I could not feel as secure with less. I would choose that same course of treatment today, four years later, and it would still be advocated.

The trend now is toward less disfiguring surgery, and the pressure from many women is in that direction. Many, taking the position that doctors are "out to get them," conjure up images of surgeons gleefully wielding scalpels over their breasts, eager to create a new race of Amazons. In many cases, the battle to save the breast against all odds has ended in loss of life. I have met many women who insist on viewing this as a black-and-white issue: mastectomy on one side and lumpectomy on the other, refusing to acknowledge the many shaded areas of disease and treatment gradation in between. We, as a society, are demanding more and more immediate gratification; quick, absolute answers to complex issues. The immediate reward of saving the breast can be paid for dearly when the type of cancer would have responded more successfully to a more invasive surgical procedure. What comfort then is a quick victory? I have also met women who have, against several surgeons' warnings, continued to search until they managed to find one who would perform a lumpectomy. You can always find someone to go along with you if you look long and hard enough. These women choose to accent the successes of the treatment they seek while denying the failures. Through interviews with prominent surgeons representing the spectrum of opinion in this constantly changing field, I'll try to illuminate the pros and cons involved in each form of treatment. Though the concept is anxiety-provoking to the layperson, medical theories are not engraved in stone.

I trotted along after Dr. Robert Somers, an energetic breast surgeon and director of the breast cancer program at the Albert Einstein Medical Center in Philadelphia, as he gave me a tour of the facilities. Regretting that I had left my running shoes at home, I asked Dr. Somers whether his views on breast cancer surgery had changed drastically over the past ten years. He replied, "Ten years ago, I would have said mastectomy *only*, but I have learned. The field is changing all the time. As Pogo says, 'I have met the enemy and he is us.' If we don't adapt to changes, we will become our own worst enemy. But ask me again in 1999 what I think."

When I first realized that it would be impossible to write about reconstruction thoroughly without including a brief discussion of the reason for it all, mastectomy, I made an appointment to talk to Dr. David Habif, at Columbia-Presbyterian Medical Center in New York City. So much had changed in thinking about breast cancer in the four years since my own mastectomy that I needed a rundown to bring me up to date. I suppose, too, that I needed to be reassured once again that I had not been a candidate for lumpectomy. Recently many mastectomized women have confided in me that they have begun to feel a subtle, unspoken pressure from lumpectomy patients, the message being that if they hadn't rushed into mastectomy, they could have saved their breast as others have done. So, on behalf of my "sisters," I embarked on a lengthy lesson on the diagnosis and treatment of breast cancer. Believe me, it's complex and emotionally charged. After attending a symposium on breast cancer during which the exchange of theories became particularly heated, I commented to a surgeon acquaintance on the ability of the subject to generate emotional turmoil on all sides. He smiled knowingly. "Yes, and you get particularly emotional when your statistics aren't good."

David Habif is a gentle, twinkly-eyed father figure of a man. I sat across from him at his desk, I with my note pad and tape recorder, he with his white-coated elbows resting on the arms of his chair, index fingers pressed to his lips, his hands making an A shape. A child's rhyme floated in and out of my mind, "Here is the church, here is the steeple, open the door and see the people."

He began by describing a candidate for lumpectomy: one with a small tumor, less than 2 centimeters in diameter, in the lower lateral quadrant, or lower outer quarter, of the breast, with no palpable spread of disease to the lymph nodes. He explained that with larger tumors the local recurrence rate is much higher and mastectomy should be performed. After a lumpectomy, however, if there is a local recurrence, secondary surgery (mastectomy) would be necessary. Dr. Habif stressed repeatedly that lumpectomy-radiation is still an experimental form of treatment. The five- and seven-year figures are interesting but not yet conclusive. With the use of radiation, he warns, you may have to go to fifteen- or twenty-year follow-up to be sure that the treatment itself does not give rise to further cancer. "When you're talking about a cure for cancer, you have to have a minimum ten-year follow-up on lumpectomy-radiation for all patients. With mastectomy, we know exactly what it is and what it has been. We don't have the same history yet with lumpectomy and radiation. So far, there is still a higher local recurrence rate with the newer form of treatment."

He explained that with a lumpectomy for malignancy the

surgeon must always remove the axillary lymph nodes as well. He cautioned, "Remember, the only purpose of radiation is to save the breast and prevent local recurrence; it has nothing to do with cure rate statistics. Women must understand that radiation has nothing to do with survival. Its sole purpose is to save the breast." He stressed that if there is a spread of disease to the lymph nodes after lumpectomy, then adjuvant chemotherapy must be given for the *body* as well as radiation for the breast. (Adjuvant chemotherapy is that which is administered as an extra precaution, assuming that the malignancy has been surgically excised, to ensure the eradication of any wandering cancer cells in the rest of the body. This has been demonstrated to substantially reduce the rate of disease recurrence.) So lumpectomy-radiation procedures are not curative alone if there is cancer elsewhere in the system.

When I mentioned this to Dr. Somers, he argued that the higher local recurrence rate with lumpectomy-radiation in the ten-year figures is thus explained: the last patient treated to have been included in the ten-year follow-up statistics would have been in 1974, when there was no chemotherapy. Drug therapy has been available only since 1975–76. Surgeons weren't removing the nodes at that time because there was no way to treat them if they were positive. They just treated the breast with X rays. Dr. Somers therefore claims that if you performed a mastectomy at that time, removing all of the breast tissue, of course you had a much lower rate of local recurrence than if you only removed part of the tissue, as in lumpectomy. This is why he places such importance on the figures for the past several years since chemotherapy has been available. He also stresses that chemotherapy treatment should start within four weeks postsurgery because the immune system is not working well and so at that point the cancer is growing quickly. His theory ("Remember, it's just a theory") is that perhaps surgery interferes with the body's immune surveillance system, which would normally keep cancer cells under control.

Oncologists interviewed, such as Dr. George Hyman of

Columbia-Presbyterian Medical Center, state, however, that their patients receiving radiation treatment do not respond as well to chemotherapy as others. The disadvantage in combining chemotherapy and radiation is that the latter can permanently suppress the patient's white blood count, which is used to calculate the most effective administration of chemotherapeutic agents. If the white count is artificially suppressed, the dosage received can be considered less than adequate for disease control. When I mentioned to Dr. Hyman that radiation therapists suggest using a granulocyte count rather than a white cell count to calculate dosage for those patients, his response was "That is just a question of semantics. The granulocytes are white cells which fight infection, but you must take the whole white count in order to arrive at the granulocyte count." He also stressed that adequate pathology is that which is done on at least twenty-five nodes, although the number of lymph nodes varies widely from person to person.

Dr. Habif made the point that radiation has been demonstrated as leading to the development of subsequent cancers. Women who were exposed to the atomic blast in Hiroshima as well as those given fluoroscopy treatment for tuberculosis had cancers develop twenty to twenty-five years after exposure. All radiotherapists interviewed agreed that there is an unknowable side effect of radiation for breast cancer. Dr. Somers and others argue that lower-dosage X-ray treatment over a long period of time is the problem in the Hiroshima and fluoroscopy cases, not the short-period high dose used in treating breast cancer. He counsels his patients, in helping them make the treatment decision, "It's a balanced scale; on the one side you have lumpectomy-radiation, and on the other side you have mastectomy and reconstruction. In both you end up with a breast."

In order to provide tumor control in a lumpectomized breast, Dr. Habif equates adequate radiation dosage to 12,000 to 15,000 chest X rays. Also, he claims that few radiotherapists can achieve really good cosmetic results. Harvard Medical School's Joint Center for Radiation Therapy reports that 25 percent of irradiated breasts are not cosmetically satisfactory. So, in many cases, women can end up with a misshapen lumpectomized breast, a scar from removal of the lymph nodes, and a discolored, hardened breast caused by radiotherapy.

Dr. Somers reports that, in an attempt to minimize the "dimpling" effect of a lumpectomy, he does not suture the two sides of the wound together. Instead, he leaves the area open, allowing it to fill in naturally. This interferes less with the breast shape and produces a better cosmetic result.

Most women assume that, with lumpectomy and radiation, they will come away with pretty much the same breast they had before. Some will be lucky, but unfortunately, that isn't always the case and there are still the increased risks of long-term radiation effects and higher local-recurrence rates. Cosmetically, and in terms of long-range health factors, they may be better off with a mastectomy and a reconstructed breast.

I visited Dr. Jerome Urban of Memorial Sloan-Kettering Cancer Center, a leading proponent of mastectomy. He feels that, with careful, thorough primary surgery, the patient with early disease has an excellent cure rate even without chemotherapy. Dr. Urban is a white-haired, soft-spoken man with a gentle manner who said, at the outset, that he was pleased to have the opportunity to dispel the myth that surgeons who perform mastectomy are sadists, doing their best to hurt people. He feels that surgeons are being beaten over the head on both sides: on one by the public, and on the other by physicians such as the group at the National Institutes of Health in Washington, D.C., who claim that what you do with primary surgery doesn't matter. If the patient has positive lymph node involvement, these physicians say that she must have chemotherapy to halt the disease spread, but Urban feels that chemotherapy isn't that good. He added that there are also no long-term results on chemotherapy as yet. His results with careful surgery and careful removal of the lymph nodes were better at the five-year follow-up than were those with patients who had had mastectomy and chemotherapy. (Once again I remind myself that the use of chemotherapy for breast cancer has been relatively recent, so this comparison may not be totally valid yet.)

The NIH thesis is that everybody with breast cancer has systemic disease. Urban feels that his figures, without chemotherapy, prove to the contrary. "If the NIH is accurate, then everyone should be on aggressive chemotherapy and there would be no point to surgery." He feels that there is no really effective chemotherapy for breast cancer, unlike certain other types of cancer. The opposing argument is that it doesn't matter what you do with your primary therapy because chemotherapy will take care of it. He considers that "absolute nonsense" and complains that "the NIH meets once a year, by invitation only, to review their material, and they invite only people who go along with what they want to hear. They have tremendous control over the whole field. Those who run the meeting and finance it decide who they want to have come. If you do go and argue with them, you never get invited back, and if someone applies for a grant that they oppose, they never get it."

Dr. Urban went on to deal with the argument of the radiotherapists who claim they do just as well as the surgeons in terms of results. In one instance, at a medical meeting, he listened to a speaker/radiotherapist claiming very low figures for local recurrence after lumpectomy and X ray and using a chart as demonstration. None of the figures were over 7 percent. Dr. Urban showed me the latest ten-year figures from Dr. Calle at the Curie Institute in Paris regarding lumpectomy-radiation follow-up.

To understand these statistics, it's necessary to clarify some basic terms used in discussing the disease. Stage I breast cancer is defined as a tumor less than two centimeters in diameter with no spread of disease to the lymph nodes. Stage II is a tumor two to five centimeters in diameter and/or involvement of the lymph nodes. For example, a woman having a one centimeter tumor and any nodal involvement is still considered a Stage II patient, as is a woman with a five centimeter tumor and no spread to the nodes. Stage III constitutes gross evidence of disease, such as a tumor over five centimeters, invasion of the muscle and skin, and enlarged, diseased lymph nodes.

The figures from Dr. Calle showed that for Stage I there was a 19 percent local recurrence rate, and for Stage II a 60 percent rate. When Dr. Urban questioned the figures on the speaker's chart, the radiotherapist acknowledged that 7 percent was the rate of recurrence in *one* particular year, but that had never been stated at the meeting. Unfortunately, others who are enthusiastic about new findings see that chart and take it as gospel. Dr. Urban attended a meeting recently where another doctor was using the same chart to support his radiation claims.

Dr. Urban's figures on local recurrence with mastectomy only, with 44 percent of the women having positive lymph nodes, were a little under 6 percent overall for local recurrence after ten years. That broke down into 1.8 percent for Stage I patients, 7 percent for Stage II, and 13 percent for Stage III. With positive nodes, X ray was given to the peripheral nodes. Dr. Urban stated that his 1.8 percent at ten years compares favorably with the figures of the lumpectomy-radiation proponents at Harvard and Memorial of 13 percent local recurrence for Stage I at six years. The rate for the Stage II lumpectomy-radiation patients was 14 percent local recurrence. They did not include any Stage III patients in their study. Dr. Urban feels that his position is like saying there is no Santa Claus because the public wants to hear only that they don't have to give up the breast. "Right now I have about 120 patients in Memorial Hospital who are back for repeat surgery after less than adequate surgery and aggressive X-ray therapy. They should never have had those recurrences. I'm seeing this more and more and feel that these women are not going to do as well as they might have if they had thorough primary surgery. I see no reason whatsoever to diminish one's efforts to control the disease locally. With good, complete surgery, I can still get the best salvage rate even with patients with positive nodes. I give chemotherapy when I feel there is a relatively poor prognosis, but I'm afraid that it will not accomplish much except to delay the progress of the cancer."

Many oncologists, however, feel that cancer is an immune disease. Therefore, if the body did not fight the primary tumor, why should it be trusted to fight the nodal involvement without chemotherapy? How else can we handle systemic involvement at this point?

Dr. Urban states that he has even seen patients develop malignancies while on chemotherapy when the surgeon has tried to do less, hoping that the chemotherapy would take care of the disease. The patient, he feels, might have been cured if the surgery had been more thorough, but, with recurrence, her prognosis is very poor. "I hear a lot of statements made based on wishful thinking but no hard proof," he says. "More of a deal is made now about saving the breast than about killing the cancer."

He has seen some breasts which, after radiation, have become shrunken, rocklike, and discolored. The results he has seen vary tremendously. Other complications of radiation, which he demonstrated with slides, can include bone changes (fragmentation and, eventually, disintegration) and necrosis (sloughing off of skin). One slide showed the torso of a woman whose clavicle (collarbone) had disappeared and whose ribs were broken after radiation. Many of these changes do not occur until fifteen or more years after treatment. Urban feels that it is too early to say whether other cancers will develop from radiation, but he suspects that it is so. He explained that after exposure to any sort of carcinogen it takes about fifteen to twenty years for a malignancy to develop. He pointed out that the incidence of cancer in the women exposed to the atom bomb and those having fluoroscopy in the course of treatment for tuberculosis was five to nine times greater than it should have been. In the fluoroscopy cases, it always occurred in the breast where the tuberculosis was located, and in the inner half, which is not too common. In the Japanese women, cancer developed in the younger ones who were exposed rather than in the age group traditionally at high risk. This was, in both cases, fifteen to twenty years after exposure.

Dr. Urban has occasionally performed a partial mastectomy by choice. A sample case was an eighty-five-year-old woman, mentally slow, with a history of multiple heart attacks and a chance of living only another two or three years. With adequate surgery for the cancer, Dr. Urban felt that she might die on the operating table, so he took out as much disease as possible to enable her to live comfortably for two to three years.

He sees most of the women with small tumors rushing into lumpectomy now in an effort to save the breast. Physicians pushing the new approaches emphasize that this is the way to go for early breast cancer, but Urban sees a great deal of risk in that. However, "it takes a long time to show that they are making a mistake. It's difficult today to get a paper published on adequate surgery because they are only interested in the new vogue, lumpectomy, so you have very little opportunity to defend your position."

I asked him to explain the interpretation of medical statistics, since the medical consumer is often at a loss when trying to interpret data on breast cancer survival. I found (and this has been corroborated by many physicians) that it would often take me more time to determine the method of statistics gathering in a particular report than it did to read the entire paper. Dr. Urban explained that statistics used to be "crude" statistics, i.e., survival calculated by listing any patient as having died of cancer even if she had died of a coronary. The only other patients included were those alive and free of disease. Now, however, a life table is used that is a more equitable way to evaluate the effect of the cancer. In this method, if a patient dies with no evidence of disease, she is removed from the series. If she dies with disease or of a coronary but has disease, she is listed as lost to cancer. If she's living with disease, she's classified as alive with disease. She has to be alive and free of disease to be considered cured. The three categories in the life table method are: (1) alive without disease; (2) alive with disease; and (3) dead of disease. Dr. Urban stressed that it's very important to state what method of gathering is used in a paper, but often it is not mentioned. In the past, any local recurrence of cancer would be listed. Some papers cite only the patients whose first sign of recurrence was a local recurrence. That is fine, Urban says, but they must specify that fact.

In January, 1984, I attended the Annual Breast Cancer Symposium at New York University Medical Center. Dr. Arthur Holleb, Senior Vice President for Medical Affairs of the American Cancer Society, speaking on the alternatives in the care of patients with breast cancer, began by quoting Oliver Wendell Holmes, who said: "To have doubted one's principles is the mark of a civilized man." He went on to say that "in spite of opinions to the contrary, surgeons are civilized men and women, willing to look at evidence and to change when change is needed . . . progress has to do with the reinterpretation of basic ideas. I think we must always remember that a clash of doctrines and ideas is not a disaster, it's merely an opportunity. . . ."

Dr. Henry Leis of New York Medical College, Valhalla, New York, talking about the surgeon's approach to the patient, said that, when discussing the treatment options with the patient, she should be told that breast cancer can very often be multicentric (i.e., there may be multiple sites of origin of the cancer in either breast) and that partial mastectomy will leave breast tissue that is at great risk. If she is adamantly opposed to having a mastectomy, he said that it is the surgeon's responsibility to inform her of radiotherapy as an alternative treatment, with the caveat that it is still being studied to evaluate its effectiveness and safety and that there are varying reports about survival and recurrence rates, as well as complications. He cautioned that if the patient favors lumpectomy, it is the responsibility of the surgeon to explain and enumerate the risks of that procedure, as well as those of radiation, and to inform her that there are certain types, stages, and locations of cancer which, traditionally, do poorly on radiotherapy. "There are a considerable number of local and regional complications of various magnitude which must be listed, some of which are not seen for a considerable period of time after therapy . . . cosmetic appearance and functional results not infrequently are not satisfactory." Dr. Leis stressed that the patient must be fully informed of the significant number of recurrences, post-radiotherapy, that do not show up for long periods of time; when they do, a secondary mastectomy must be performed. He reported that those percentages are considerably higher than with mastectomy. The possibility of spray radiation (the scatter effect of radiation treatment) causing cancer in the opposite breast was mentioned, as well as radiation-induced cancers in other areas. These, Dr. Leis agreed, can develop over a twenty-to-thirty-year period. The patient, he said, must be informed of all of these factors; that is the responsibility of the surgeon.

Rose Kushner, the director of the Breast Cancer Advisory Center, in Kensington, Maryland, feels that "if a woman goes to a mastectomy surgeon first, she gets a mastectomy. If she goes to a radiation therapist first, she gets radiation." She stated that the American Cancer Society should be involved in pretreatment breast cancer counseling and strongly urged that there be an international organization of trained people to do this type of counseling. In addressing the subject of radiation, she said, "Radiation, while a conservation procedure, is not a conservative procedure. Five to six thousand rads to the breast is certainly not conservative. . . . ASTRO [the American Society for Therapeutic Radiation Oncology] has under two thousand members. Of those, there are not two hundred who have the appropriate training and equipment to provide good treatment of the intact breast." She went on to advise women that if they don't have the money to go where there is radiation expertise, they would be well advised to have a mastectomy and reconstruction. She reported seeing burned breasts, lymphedema (swelling of tissues), and brachial neuropathy (nerve damage in the radiated region) caused by poor radiation. She also stated that many third-party insurance carriers do not pay for radiotherapy, while most are now paying for reconstruction.

Dr. Samuel Hellman, physician-in-chief at Memorial Sloan-Kettering Cancer Center in New York, is a proponent of lumpectomy-radiation. He terms this treatment "preservative" surgery in that it preserves the breast. He is an articulate, confident man, considerably younger than many of his colleagues at the symposium. He stated that the goal of his treatment is to eradicate all disease in the local area and in the region but preserve the breast. He also pointed out that his is an evolving technique. "We try to learn how to do it, and if one learns how to do it, one changes along the way."

Dr. Hellman's treatment plan with radiotherapy consists of a dose to the breast of a maximum of 5,000 rads and a minimum of 4,600. Added to that is an implant dose of approximately 2,200 rads, amounting to more than 7,000 rads altogether. The implant dose is in the form of iridium needles in nylon tubing inserted into the breast. This dose also goes to the underlying normal tissues, which he terms quite acceptable. The small defects where the iridium implant needles were inserted will still be visible a couple of years later, he reports.

Dr. Hellman acknowledged that it is still too soon to talk about survival with this technique, but he finds the statistics encouraging. He reports follow-up figures after six years of 4 percent local recurrence for Stage I patients and 13 percent for Stage II. The classification of those patients is based on clinical, not pathological, staging, the difference being that clinical staging is judged by the surgeon's palpation while pathological staging is the result of microscopic examination of tissue in the laboratory. In Hellman's study, even if the patients had axillary node samplings that turned out to be pathologically positive, if their nodes had been clinically negative they were classified as Stage I. The survival was 92 percent for Stage I and 83 percent for Stage II at six years. It is Dr. Habif's assertion, however, that local recurrence figures traditionally increase with time, so it is possible that the ten-year figures on lumpectomy-radiation will not be as good.

Dr. Hellman states, "The purpose of this treatment is to give the woman a good cosmetic result. The doctor's role, in my judgment, is to put the patients back to where they were before they had the disease. A pre-morbid status in breast cancer is closest achieved when the woman looks and feels as she did before the lump." He went on to report that about half of the local recurrences occur within five years and that some of these recurrences can be salvaged. Thirty of the women in his study who had local recurrences were then treated by mastectomy and had a 50 percent likelihood of being cured. He cautioned that "for partial mastectomy without radiation, there is tremendous local breast relapse in a very short time. That is not a viable option if you believe that the purpose of treatment is to reduce local recurrence to the smallest possible number. I conclude that radiation and limited surgery for resection of the primary [tumor] and determination of axillary node status is an alternative which is acceptable for the treatment of breast cancer. The technique, if done properly, will give us good cosmetic results, high local control, and this alternative is comparable to surgery for the time it has been studied. The difference is that we haven't got as much long-term data on it. That's the uncertainty. The risk is not with the data we have, but I can't give patients twenty-year data when the patients haven't been followed for twenty years. If patients accept that as an uncertainty, then I believe that this is a viable option. If I thought it was going to go poorly, then obviously I couldn't recommend it. There aren't any data to suggest it. But that's again a crystal ball."

When questioned about the long-term cancer risks of radiotherapy, Dr. Hellman said, "I think that's a major question that needs to be answered. My crystal ball is just a crystal ball." He elaborated by observing that whereas most of the local recurrences occur in the first ten years, most radiation-induced cancers occur after that. However, his feeling is that breast cancer patients are not the group traditionally at risk, as are the nuclear attack victims or the tuberculosis sufferers, pointing out that those women received low-dosage radiation applied over a long period, whereas his patients receive a high dosage over a short period. There may, however, be a problem in the opposite breast, he acknowledged, which is the recipient of lower scatter doses from treatment of the other side. He mentioned that the high incidence of breast cancer in the long-term radiation study groups was in women under thirty-five and summed up by saying, "I don't think our group is at much risk, but that's the extent of my crystal ball. We'll just have to wait and see."

It would appear, after investigating all approaches to breast cancer treatment, that everybody's got his (or her) own "religion." Each physician believes strongly in his own protocol. Therefore, if you are in doubt, two or three opinions are in order, and you should be as fully informed as possible about the benefits and drawbacks of each form of treatment. Is the treatment you would like to choose the best one for your long-term health profile? For your peace of mind? Remember, we're talking about life here—not just next month or next year. I don't know about you, but I like as few visible question marks in that area as possible.

Another puzzling aspect of treatment is the manner in which the pathology is handled in different hospitals. I had the naïve impression that pathology in one laboratory would be the same as in another. I did learn that whereas in most hospitals the pathology report was available in a couple of days after removal of the breast tissue and nodes, it can take anywhere from two weeks to one month in a hospital that conducts multistaged pathologic diagnosis. I waited two and a half weeks for my results and have often wondered if the two cancer cells in that one lymph node would have been detected in a more cursory examination. Would I have been given the green light in terms of chemotherapy anywhere else? And what would that have meant in terms of recurrence for me? Of course, there's the explanation of my body being able to handle a microscopic metastasis by itself. Perhaps, *à la* Dr. Somers's hypothesis, the surgery interfered with the immune surveillance, my body's burglar alarm. But if that were the case, then chemotherapy became my watchdog. What I do know is that I have many women acquaintances who are still here years after mastectomy with early detection, whereas I don't know any who have the history yet to prove likewise with lumpectomy-radiation. No one hopes more than I that they will be here years from now to prove the newer theories; I have a beloved daughter, sister, stepdaughters, etc., etc. The one point on which *everyone* agrees is that early detection is of critical, lifesaving importance. So whatever your choice of surgery, have it done early, and if you can't live with a gamble or lumpectomy is not appropriate for you, then consider reconstruction after mastectomy.

6

Is Reconstruction for You?

In order for each postmastectomy woman to be able to make an educated decision for or against breast reconstruction, she must be presented with the spectrum of choices and the techniques involved in each. A formidable array, at first glance, but it's a bit like reading all the steps involved in the preparation of a seven-course haute cuisine banquet before even walking into the kitchen; one step at a time is a lot easier.

Postmastectomy chests, as we now know, do not all look the same. They vary, depending upon the extent of the cancer surgery and the skill of the surgeon. In the early days of reconstruction, women who underwent any procedure more complex than a simple or modified radical mastectomy could not hope for rehabilitative surgery. With the development of new techniques, that has all been changed, and now even the most radically altered chests can be rebuilt. The reconstructive process there may be more complicated and lengthier than others, but it can be done. Even if you feel that reconstruction may not be for you, you owe it to yourself to be as fully informed as possible, for only then can you make a decision based on accumulated knowledge rather than on myth.

Many breast surgeons are now routinely suggesting reconstruction for their appropriate mastectomy patients. There are still, however, many older, conservative holdouts. In that case, you must make known your interest in the procedure. The most important point of all—and I cannot stress it too strongly—is that no one must feel under pressure to reconstruct; the motivation must come from within, not from without. It is one of the most personal decisions you'll ever make, and you have many areas of control therein. You can choose to reconstruct or not to. You can also put off the decision and see how you feel about it one, two, or several years from now. Remember, it is your choice and you are entitled to the privilege of making it. What is comforting for another woman may not be right for you. Ultimately, do what will make you, and only you, feel best, and allow other women their choices as well. We all make our own private accommodations to the issue of breast cancer, and as my musician friend would say, "Hey, man, whatever gets you through the night. . . ."

In the years since my own reconstruction, the range of techniques and options has increased considerably. The choice of procedure is based on the degree of primary surgery as well as on psychological need. I'll enumerate the major options here and go on to explain them further by way of my interviews with expert surgeons.

1. Simple Implant Insertion

Appropriate for subcutaneous mastectomy, a prophylactic procedure occasionally recommended for women at very high risk. In this type of surgery, the breast tissue has been removed, leaving the muscle, skin, and nipple-areola intact. Simple and modified radical mastectomies leaving ample skin for coverage also qualify for simple implant insertion. A simple mastectomy removes breast tissue, nipple-areola, and varying amounts of breast skin, leaving the chest muscle and lymph nodes. A modified radical, also known as a total mastectomy with axillary dissection, saves the chest muscle but removes the breast tissue, breast skin, nipple-areola, and lymph nodes.

2. Expanders

These are temporary expanding implants for simple or modified mastectomies where the skin is very tight and/or very thin. After the expanders have stretched the skin, they are replaced by a permanent implant.

3. Latissimus Dorsi Flap (latissimus dorsi myodermal flap)

Appropriate for radical mastectomies, to replace the pectoral muscle with one from the back, this requires the use of an implant to create a breast mound. Radical mastectomies, also called Halsted radicals, remove the breast tissue, breast skin, nipple-areola, chest muscles, and underarm lymph nodes. The latissimus dorsi procedure creates an apparent back scar.

4. RAM (Rectus abdominis myodermal flap)

This is used for modified radical or radical mastectomies. In modified radicals, it is used to re-create a breast mound without the need for an implant. In radical mastectomies, it replaces the pectoral muscle with abdominal muscle, creating the entire breast mound with abdominal tissue. The RAM creates apparent abdominal scarring.

5. Gluteal Free Flap (Superior Gluteal Microvascular Free Flap)

This is used for radical or modified radical mastectomies. For modified radical patients, it re-creates a breast mound without an implant. In radicals, it replaces the pectoral (chest) muscle with a muscle flap from the upper portion of the buttock, creating a breast mound with buttock tissue. The donor site has apparent scarring.

Immediate reconstruction is now performed in all of the above methods with the exception of the gluteal free flap. In each of these procedures, if nipple-areola grafts are desired, they constitute a separate surgical procedure performed on an outpatient basis. The reconstructive procedures listed range in length from less than one hour for simple implants to approximately five or six hours for the most complex. At present, the latissimus dorsi takes three to four hours at best, the RAM even longer, and the gluteal free flap longest by one to two hours. These operating times are increased with less experienced surgeons. Recuperation is also lengthier with the more complex reconstructive procedures, sometimes requiring up to ten days in hospital.

Over the past year I have interviewed many cancer surgeons, plastic surgeons, and oncologists, as well as attending symposiums on breast cancer and reconstruction in an attempt to present here as broad a spectrum of technique and approach as possible in this constantly evolving field. It is difficult for the layperson to consider surgery an art; we so desperately want it to be an absolute science. The reality is that opinions and techniques vary enormously and your education to them is critical. Reconstruction is one of the newest innovations in the art of surgery, and the rest of this chapter should provide a comprehensive view of the current state of this new art form.

One helpful piece of advice comes from Dr. Robert DeVito, the Northwestern Regional Coordinator for the American Society of Plastic and Reconstructive Surgeons, who suggests that if the cancer surgeon's response to reconstruction is along the lines of "Don't be so narcissistic" or "You're lucky to be alive" or "Leave well enough alone," the patient should walk right out of the office and head for the next doctor on her list. There is nothing quite so infuriating for a mastectomized woman as to be told what her emotional needs should be. It reminds me of a friend who, during a rather heated discussion, once said to me, "You can tell me how my actions affect you, but don't ever presume to tell me what's going on in *my* head!" I never tried it again.

Enlightened breast cancer surgeons expressed nothing but encouragement for the patient. Dr. Arthur Holleb said that breast reconstruction is a "very personal choice by the woman herself" and that "plastic surgeons are to be congratulated on their remarkable abilities in reconstructing a normal appearance." It was also encouraging to hear his comment that "the input of the patient is extremely helpful."

Dr. Henry Leis advocated that the surgeon, in discussing the various types of mastectomy and the particular kind being recommended, also deal with the possibility of breast reconstruction, including the pros and cons of immediate versus delayed reconstruction. He stressed that patients be informed, however, that "while the results are very rewarding, the reconstruction does not entirely restore them to their premastectomy appearance." He reported that over one million silicone implants have been used to date.

Even though we continue to hear reports of breast surgeons resisting the concept of reconstruction, both Drs. Holleb and Leis were enthusiastic in their expressions that women should be made aware of this opportunity. Neither man, though vital and energetic, appeared to have begun practice yesterday, so it would appear that the reluctance of older surgeons to recommend reconstruction to women is not universal by any means.

I talked to Dr. David Habif about reconstruction from the point of view of the cancer surgeon. He is very encouraging to women about to undergo mastectomy and always suggests plastic surgery except in cases where the disease is quite advanced and the tumor is large. Age is not a determining factor. He suggests that if reconstruction is not mentioned by the surgeon, the patient say, "I have reconstruction in mind and I'm relying on you to tell me when." Dr. Habif also told me that he has never seen a recurrence of cancer due to reconstruction, which is a fear voiced by some surgeons and patients.

When I asked if there were any modifications that a cancer surgeon might make in technique to facilitate reconstruction, he replied, "Most breast surgeons do not do cancer surgery with reconstruction in mind; the primary goal is always to get the disease out. However, with a large breast and a small intraductal cancer [a cancer originating in the milk ducts], I leave as much of the breast pocket as possible and try not to take a large amount of skin." He believes that the ideal mastectomy incision is a horizontal or transverse one, next best would be the oblique, and the least attractive would be the vertical incision, which would have to start high up at the collarbone. He feels that any of these could be reopened to insert the implant, or another incision could be made under the breast (an inframammary incision). If the tumor is large or sitting on or invading the pectoral muscle, then the muscle must be removed (a radical mastectomy). At first surgeons attempted to save and store the nipple, to be used in reconstructing the breast. This is now discouraged because, in many cases, the nipple ducts can also be cancer-prone.

Dr. Habif went on to explain that, with regard to discussing reconstruction, when the surgeon feels the axilla (lymph nodes in the armpit) before surgery, his error in predicting a metastasis (spread of cancer) to the nodes is 30 percent either way; i.e., in 100 women thought to have negative nodal involvement, 30 will turn out to be positive. The preoperative judgment is called clinical diagnosis, but when the removed nodes are examined in the laboratory, that constitutes a pathological diagnosis. Microscopic involvement cannot be detected by the surgeon's palpation before the operation. Dr. Habif therefore feels he can't discuss reconstruction that specifically until he knows whether the patient will require chemotherapy. In that case, he recommends waiting until after chemotherapy for reconstruction. The course of therapy should begin as soon after surgery as possible, and surgery during chemotherapy is not recommended unless absolutely necessary.

We also talked about insurance coverage for breast reconstruction. Dependent (pendulous) breasts often require reduction surgery (mammoplasty) or lifting (mastopexy). Small breasts may require augmentation to achieve a match. Insurance companies can balk at that, making the assumption that it is a cosmetic, rather than rehabilitative, procedure. Dr. Habif emphasized that the aim of reconstruction is to achieve a match of the two breasts. Often you cannot achieve that goal without surgery on the opposite side because there isn't enough skin on the mastectomy side. Companies should pay for the reduction because the aim is the complete rehabilitation of the patient. If chemotherapy is not prescribed, three to six months is the advised waiting period after mastectomy for reconstructive surgery. Dr. Habif feels that there are no complications from mastectomy that would interfere with reconstruction and that a plastic surgeon should be present at a mastectomy only if performing a simultaneous reconstructive procedure.

Dr. Randolph H. Guthrie, Jr., a plastic surgeon affiliated with New York Hospital, is an articulate man with an engaging sense of humor. A taller, saner-looking version of Jack Nicholson, he set aside a rare, patient-free morning to acquaint me with the intricacies of breast reconstruction. He was so thorough and used such layperson language in his explanations that, after two hours, I felt qualified for at least a Ph.D. on the subject. The interview was held in his elegantly furnished new townhouse-office, so tastefully decorated and discreetly lit that, were it not for the two secretaries working behind a partition on the far wall, I would have expected a hostess to appear announcing the serving of luncheon. A curving staircase in the outer entry led to the family's private quarters, and we were visited temporarily by a regal black-and-white Persian cat who sat watching us with an air of ownership, her tiny kitten playing "cat and mouse" with us from behind the sofa. Workmen continued to put finishing touches on the suite of offices as we talked, their drilling and the phone's ringing providing the accompaniment to our conversation.

Dr. Guthrie performs breast surgery exclusively, almost all of it reconstruction, and is the person with the greatest longevity in that specialty. He performs four or five hundred reconstruction procedures each year. In 1971 he and Dr. Reuven Snyderman published the first paper on the subject in the modern era. In 1976 he published the second paper, and in between, to his knowledge, there hadn't been anything else written on the technique. He feels that now, in the rush to publish, the field has gotten a little "way out." Other types of approaches, now heralded as great new discoveries, had been discovered while he and his colleagues were working at New York Hospital and Memorial Sloan-Kettering Cancer Center. However, they didn't even report them because the techniques were found to be unsatisfactory. His opinion is that people are reporting unfortunate things under the academic pressure of "publish or perish," without always considering the patient's best interests.

Dr. Guthrie believes that one should pick from among the spectrum of available reconstructive procedures, depending upon what the patient has to start with. He is firm in stating that the most benign procedure is the one that should always be used, and that one should not undertake large procedures simply for the sake of proving that they can be done when patients don't need them. The simplest procedures, he says, give the best results. "Once we start to move to the extended procedures, the results become inferior. The simplest method is to take an implant, put it under the tissues of the chest wall at whatever depth, and leave it. That takes from forty to sixty minutes and still produces the best results." He sees more women seeking breast reconstruction now, but is not sure that it indicates more cancer at a younger age, even though that is his impression. It is the younger women who are more interested in being reconstructed. Women are also learning to be aware of the possibility of breast cancer earlier, detecting it sooner, and then reconstructing. More women, Dr. Guthrie says, are beginning to demand reconstruction, changing the attitude of traditional surgeons, which he terms the "lucky-to-be-alive syndrome."

Dr. Guthrie is of the opinion that the original surgeon should never be involved in the reconstruction and, conversely, the plastic surgeon should never be involved in the mastectomy, except in a minor advisory capacity. "The one doing the mastectomy is there to save your life, and nobody wants to die for a reconstruction. The surgeon doing the mastectomy can reach a point where, if he knew much about reconstruction—and fortunately most of them don't—he would know that, if he goes just a step further, he [the plastic surgeon] is not going to be able to do just a simple implantation reconstruction, but a four-to-five-hour procedure. The first priority is the life . . . so a cancer surgeon should never be on that kind of fence. He should not be thinking about how he's going to put her back together again. There's a whole range from good to bad in surgeons, as in anything else. That's just inherent in the spectrum of talent. By and large, I don't think the extent of the mastectomy is dependent upon the skill of the surgeon. It may be dependent somewhat on his judgment, which might be bad. He may have taken off more than he needed. There's the old school that says if you don't take off everything you can see and smell, you haven't done the proper job."

Dr. Guthrie went on to cite some things which could be done quite easily during mastectomy without jeopardizing the safety of the patient and which would facilitate a better cosmetic result in reconstruction. In his view, the scar should be oblique so that no part of it shows inside the brassiere line. When it is completely horizontal and comes across the midline, it's visible in the V of a dress or bathing suit. The surgeon can stop that scar short of where it shows, but, very often, Dr. Guthrie has seen surgeons bring it across and onto the other breast. He told me that three areas of the body are prone to scar heavily, ropily, and red: the shoulders, the deltoid region (the outer, topmost area of the upper arm), and the triangle over the sternum, or breastbone. The mastectomy scar, if over the sternum, can sabotage the most magnificent reconstruction, and in Dr. Guthrie's view there is no reason for that. The easiest way to avoid it is to make the scar oblique because, no matter how long it is, unless it comes out the bottom of the brassiere, it can't reach the midsternum. If the surgeon starts out with a horizontal scar and then has to extend it, you're stuck, whereas if he has to extend the oblique line, he can still go down a little farther and be out of the way. If the cancer is in the upper part of the breast, it's more difficult to get up so high with a horizontal incision, whereas, with an oblique, there is more flexibility.

Dr. Guthrie then described the four levels of implantation:

1. The implant can be put just under the fat (subcutaneous).
2. The pectoralis muscle can be split so that some of it is in front of the implant and some behind.
3. The implant can go completely behind the pectoralis muscle.
4. It can go completely behind both the pectoralis and the upper abdominal muscle, which is attached to the pectoralis at its bottom edge.

Dr. Guthrie demonstrated, on himself, the path of the pectoralis muscle as it sweeps obliquely down from the armpit toward the middle of the chest. He explained that an implant that is just under the pectoralis muscle has its lower outer quarter uncovered. If the surgeon wants it all covered with muscle, he has to pick up the serratus muscle, which comes around from the side. That and the pectoralis muscle both attach to the fifth rib, so if they are both picked up, they're in effect attached to each other, which provides a continuum of muscle having a thin strip of gristle tissue between the two. That muscle is called the "serratus flap," but, technically, it is really not. In fact, the serratus muscle arises at the same place as the external oblique muscle, which swings forward and goes to the midline, the rectus. Since both the serratus and the external oblique arise at the same place, if they are picked up together they intermingle. If the surgeon goes very far to the side when creating the implant pocket, he will indeed pick up some serratus fibers, but most are fibers in the front, which are actually external oblique. The reason for all the confusion is that the surgeons who did the operation originally didn't know their anatomy very well, so they mistakenly named it the "serratus flap." In fact, it is really the external oblique muscle for most of the front and then, at the lower middle of the implant pocket, the rectus muscle (the one that goes down the center of the abdomen). So this deep insertion can actually involve three muscles, which Dr. J. W. Little in Washington appropriately dubbed a "brassiere" of muscle. In Dr. Guthrie's experience, the more tissue covering the implant, the less satisfactory the final appearance. There are several reasons for that, in his judgment:

1. The bulkier the tissue over the implant, the less discreet the final result; too much tissue blends the implant out on its sides, tending to flatten it.
2. If the muscle is on top of the implant, when it contracts with movement it can flatten the implant and, in some cases, make it "dance" or twitch. In twitching, the whole muscle contracts at once and makes the implant ride up. Dr. Guthrie has many patients who were reconstructed elsewhere for whom he has had to alleviate this problem. This can be effected, to a large extent, by releasing the muscle where it inserts on the middle and the bottom. Because it cannot be released totally, the problem can be ameliorated but not completely eliminated.
3. In Dr. Guthrie's experience, there is much more risk of bleeding when the surgeon goes into the muscle, and that can be a very severe problem. He feels that it is one of the prime precursors of hard implants, a common complication of breast reconstruction. The blood clots and forms a framework into which scar tissue grows, and it is tight scar tissue that causes hard implants.
4. The principal problem with putting the implant under the

pectoral muscle, with or without the serratus, is that the muscles are meant to glide on the chest, freely attached to the ribs, with a very fine tissue-paper kind of connection. But there is little, if any, connection between the back side of the muscle and the ribs. When your arm moves up and down, the muscle must be able to move several inches. Once the space behind it is invaded, the muscle heals back except where the implant is separating it from the ribs. The muscle scars tightly where it heals and this can result, very often, in symptoms of being trapped, of limited arm motion; and if a sudden movement pulls the muscle, it can rip the scar tissue, resulting in severe pain for a few days followed by soreness for several months. That can give rise to hesitation about shoulder movement and can result in permanent limitation. This occurs in extreme cases, however. I and many other women have had submuscular implants without experiencing those difficulties.

The above points argue, in Guthrie's view, against putting the implant too deep, even though he agrees that depth provides protection for the implant. The other extreme is that when the tissues overlying the implant are too thin, it can erode itself out. This is termed "extrusion" of the implant. The problems with trapped implants, however, can be accepted and corrected for the most part, but extrusion cannot be. The decision on depth must be made in conjunction with the patient, since she must understand that there may be a price to pay for not inserting the implant deeper. Dr. Guthrie says that he and the patient may frequently decide to go deeper than just under the fat because the implant won't stay in place there and will appear misshapen. If the patient insists on subcutaneous insertion and he doesn't think it will stay there, he won't perform the operation. There are, though, some patients for whom that will work. By and large, with a small variable, the fat must be about 8 millimeters (¼–⅜ of an inch) thick before it can be trusted to protect the implant.

In the great majority of cases, Dr. Guthrie splits the pectoral muscle, which avoids the problems of the implant being inserted deep into the muscle and scarring itself to the chest wall, but still gives a great deal of implant protection. Splitting the muscle, he feels, is almost as good as having the whole muscle in front because even a thin layer of muscle carries an enormous blood supply. Poor blood supply is the whole basis for erosion, so if the blood supply is adequate, the implant will not erode. With 75 percent of the simple implantation procedures, Dr. Guthrie advocates putting them in to about one-third the depth of the muscle. He explained further: "You normally cannot split muscle because it's so floppy that you simply cannot separate one part from another, but in the case of mastectomy, the front side of the muscle is scarred to the back side of the fat, so that it wants to cling to it. So you just scrape the muscle away. You don't scrape too efficiently, so that a large part of it remains stuck to the fat; it's hard to get off. People will say that it's impossible to do that, and my reply is that you could not normally do it, but after mastectomy you can because it's fixed in place. Then they try it and realize that it's easy. I like to put an implant in as superficially as possible commensurate with safety. Many people think I insert all implants subcutaneously. I would prefer to do that if I could, but 75 percent or more of the time I cannot. Actually, I probably don't put any more than 7–10 percent in subcutaneously, if that many. Those look the best, though."

I then asked what sort of incision he favors for the implant insertion. He explained that he never goes back through the mastectomy wound because that is the place where the maximum amount of pressure from the implant's stretching of the skin will take place. Quite a bit of skin is removed in the mastectomy, and in the interim between mastectomy and reconstruction the skin lies flat on the chest. If all of the skin had been left, there would be a big bag of skin hanging on the chest. The remaining skin must stretch in order to get back that breast shape. As in pregnancy, the skin has an amazing capacity to stretch, but the stretching takes time. When an implant is first inserted, it is usually a bit flat and too round, like half a sphere rather than a teardrop breast shape. Together, the push of the implant and gravity make the skin stretch the way it would over a normal breast. If the mastectomy wound is reopened, then all of this stretching would be taking place against a new wound which is also quite thin, having had a good deal of subcutaneous fat scraped off it.

When I asked why so much of the fat must be scraped off, he explained that the breast is not a smooth but a fuzzy ball sending out tendrils of breast tissue into the surrounding fat, so most breast surgeons feel that they should take a good deal of that fat to be sure they've removed all those little fibers of breast tissue. Normally, a mastectomy closure is done in one layer, since there's usually not enough fat left to put in a varied layer of stitches. If that wound is reopened to gain access to the pocket underneath, the closure can't be very strong and there will be a great deal of pressure against it. If the implant were to be put in superficially, just under the skin, Dr. Guthrie warns that it would surely come through the incision. The surgeon, therefore, would be committed to putting it under the muscle, and because of the approach it would have to be under all the muscle. The only way to split the muscle would be to catch it on its edge at the bottom. He compared coming through the mastectomy wound and looking at the muscle to looking at the center of a pancake from the top. You can't get around and look at the edge of it. You can do that only by going in below the muscle at the bottom edge. So the surgeon has to actually penetrate the muscle, open up the space behind it, put the implant in, close the muscle for the first layer of protection, and then close the skin. That will usually protect the implant from extrusion. It produces the problems of a submuscular implantation, but the skin is still under the same kind of pressure. It could open up and reveal muscle, a thoroughly unappealing thought. If it doesn't open up, it can spread to be a wide scar and not look as good.

The worst of it is that one cannot gain proper access to the lower part of the pocket to release the muscle. That would present all the problems of a submuscular implantation, and often the implant will not stay down where it is supposed to stay. That occurs because the muscle, where it inserts below and particularly to the middle, inserts at a zero angle. When an implant is put in, it opens that angle to make the pocket. When the muscle contracts, it wants to close the angle, and a contracting muscle has tremendous leverage. It wants to push the implant out of the corner. If that muscle cannot be cut at its point of insertion, then there is no way to get rid of this pushing problem. The most common defect after a noninframammary (not under the breast) approach is a superiorly and laterally displaced implant. In other words, it sort of migrates toward the shoulder. It only has to move out of position half an inch to look strange. For instance, in a bathing suit, one side would look as if it were riding uphill. Dr. Guthrie maintains that the under-the-breast approach "fixes you right where you want to be." Even with the risk of going in through the mastectomy incision, I remember wanting very badly to avoid more scarring. However, the inframammary incision fades and eventually looks like a shadow in the natural curve under the breast.

Dr. Guthrie does not give patients any premedication before they come to the operating room. That way, they are awake enough to sit up straight on the table with their shoulders level, something very few women do after mastectomy, he informed me. I remembered having the same problem. First he takes some Polaroid pictures of the chest to aid in placement. Then he makes a mark in the crease under the normal breast, takes a ruler straight across, and marks the mastectomy side. That mark corresponds to the bottom of the normal breast where the brassiere will fit. Even with a pendulous breast, a brassiere will bring it up to the inframammary crease. He makes the incision at that mark, knowing that everything above that line has got to be surgically released. When finished, the implant has to move freely down to the incision. He starts at that incision point, cuts through the muscle there if he's going deep, and clears it to the side to avoid an "hourglass" constricture halfway up. Then he knows that the implant is free all the way to the bottom.

When a patient is missing the muscle and the skin is either terribly tight or very thin, or when the scar is very tight and very thin, a more complex reconstructive procedure has to be done. In those instances, when an implant is inserted, the skin is going to be stretched so tightly that it simply isn't going to be able to hold the implant. Also, sometimes the other breast is so large and the skin on the mastectomy side so tight that it will not take a matching implant. In such cases, tissue can be brought in from somewhere else. Dr. Guthrie favors the latissimus dorsi flap, which was first developed at the turn of the century by Dr. Ignio Tansini in Italy and was used all over Europe to close massive wounds. It had ceased to be used when mastectomy became less radical. It was later rediscovered and modified for use in replacing the muscle lost in radical mastectomy today. It enabled people who could not previously be reconstructed to be rebuilt. Dr. Guthrie recalled contacting many patients who had given up hope of reconstruction and saying, "Hey, we've found a way!" He explained that the latissimus dorsi is on the back and is the mirror image of the pectoral muscle. Its virtue is that it gets its blood and nerve supply from up at the top. It can be freed up completely so that it is attached only at the top and then swung around under the skin and laid out over the chest. An island of skin can even be brought with it, sitting right on top of it, living off it like a parasite. The mastectomy scar is reopened; it will then gape like an ellipse. The elliptical island flap is put right into it. Once it is properly oriented, it fits right in. When this is done, the missing muscle has been put in along with additional skin to solve the tightness problem. The flap has then changed a radical mastectomy into a modified mastectomy. The latissimus dorsi flap will also improve the "washboard" appearance of the radical mastectomy patient's upper chest by creating a smooth approach as well as providing a surface for the implant.

Adding a stage takes time. Dr. Guthrie told me that, in the

hands of surgeons who do it all the time, the latissimus dorsi procedure takes two and a half to three hours, whereas with the average plastic surgeon it takes six. "There are some who don't care what you look like when you come in," he asserts; "they won't do anything but a latissimus dorsi flap, and that's wrong. Some of these patients had absolutely perfect chests for simple implants and were advised that they had to have a latissimus dorsi flap. If they would look better in the end, it might be a slight rationale for enduring a five-to-six-hour procedure, but they will look worse. This is just a matter of ignorance." He mentioned that insurance companies also pay a good deal more for a latissimus dorsi procedure.

We moved on to the various types of implants. Basically, there are three different kinds, having in common a silicone shell made from silicone with some added silica filler. One type is filled with silicone gel; the second is filled with saline solution (salt water), and the third is the double-lumen implant with two compartments: silicone gel in the inner lumen and saline solution in the outer. There is another type having silicone gel on the inside and a polyurethane fuzz (called meme) on the outside. The silicone gel implants were first used in breast augmentation in the 1950s. These are not to be confused with the liquid silicone injections also used in early breast augmentation, which created serious problems. In fact, Dr. Guthrie told me that, although there is some recent evidence that liquid silicone in itself may not be dangerous, it may be a catalyst for several very bad reactions that will more likely take place in its presence. On the other hand, the silicone shell is not at all dangerous because it's solid and the only way silicone travels is in microscopic form. If the shell is thoroughly baked in manufacture and doesn't have a liquid core left in it, it is perfectly safe.

In 1965 Dow Corning developed essentially the same silicone shell with gel implants used today. However, within a fairly short period, implanted breasts were becoming hard because the body encapsulated the implant with thick, heavy scar tissue. The scar tissue would shrink and force the implant into the shape of a sphere. It would also become more prominent because, as Dr. Guthrie explained, as it was forced into the sphere shape, it touched the chest only tangentially and the rest of the sphere's diameter would be sticking forward. Compressed around the sides, it looked like a mountain sitting on a plain. Also, on its top, the implant's superior surface would become convex where the breast should be concave. "Actually," Dr. Guthrie says, "talking about capsules is a misnomer. We should talk about tight capsules. A sphere of scar tissue forms around anything we put in the body. The problem is when it makes it too thick. A desirable membrane would be tissue-paper-thin. Contractile membranes are sometimes a quarter-inch thick and are like cement when you cut through them."

Steroids were then tried in the implant to avoid contracture. Steroids interfere with the production and cross-linking of proteins, which, it was hoped, would eliminate scar tissue. It eliminated the tight capsule but it also eliminated the skin, sometimes sloughing off the whole chest wall. The skin would turn blue and become so thin that the Mediterranean-blue water in the implant was visible. Exquisite, but who needed it on her chest? The steroid dose was lowered, but the reaction still happened. Between 65 and 90 percent of gel-filled implants hardened.

In the early 1970s polyurethane was put on the implant. It was thought that, because polyurethane was slightly irritating, it would cause a minimal reaction in the body, which would produce a vascular capsule, one with blood vessels in it. The other tight capsules contained no blood vessels (were avascular). A vascular capsule would not shrink because it would be normal tissue. That was true but, even though the capsule right next to the polyurethane was vascular, as the capsule got thicker, the polyurethane had no effect on it. Eventually, as it got to its thickest point, it became contractile. After a couple of years it would become rock-hard. Then the polyurethane was very difficult to remove because it was bonded and couldn't be removed under local anesthesia.

Also, after a while it was found to have migrated all around the chest, causing year-long draining sinuses, and lumps and bumps that women thought were other cancers. The implants also had seams that leaked. Toward the end of the decade they were pretty much abandoned. In 1983, the same manufacturer has brought them back with claims of marked improvement. Dr. Guthrie is doubtful and, because of bad experience, will not try them again.

Saline implants came in about 1975. Six manufacturers made the early ones. The incidence of capsule formation was a good deal lower, but (a big but) one out of three leaked. That was not harmful, since it was, after all, just salt water, but it was a little like having a flat tire on your chest. These implants were then abandoned by everyone because of that problem. However, Dr. Guthrie reports that one manufacturer, Heyer-Schulte, found out why they leaked and changed the shell composition. Formerly, even though it was a clear-walled, smooth-looking shell, microscopically it was discovered to be very abrasive, and, rubbing against itself when it wrinkled, would break and leak. They changed it to an opaque, thick-walled shell. It feels no thicker through the skin, and microscopically it's very smooth. Within six months Heyer-Schulte had the improved ones on the market, but many surgeons refused to try them again. Dr. Guthrie said that because Dow Corning refused to make them, it was assumed by many that they were still unsatisfactory. He has found the new ones to be terrific, leaking only once in four hundred times.

No one looks forward to a "flat tire," as Dr. Guthrie so aptly describes the infrequent results of a leaking saline implant. However, it is not as tragic an event as you might think and can be repaired in a very short outpatient procedure using a local anesthetic. Sue Lucas, the energetic division coordinator for the Reach to Recovery reconstruction program in Mississippi, tells of a tennis-playing friend who woke one morning to discover that one side of her bilaterally reconstructed chest was as flat as a board. Her husband, hearing a scream from the bathroom, ran to her aid. "I've lost it!" she exclaimed. "I've lost my left boob!" A couple of hours later they met her surgeon at the hospital, where he quickly replaced the deflated implant with a new one. The next day she played in a tennis tournament.

Dr. Guthrie finds the incidence of tight capsule formation to be very low, in the 10 percent range, with these saline implants. To minimize the incidence of capsular contracture, he also uses minute doses of steroids in the implant, a controversial issue among several other surgeons interviewed. He explained that when the new saline implants were first used, the incidence of tight capsule formation was nearly halved. In Canada, Dr. E. R. Parrin did extensive research studies on steroid use in the implant: tiny doses leaching out over a six-to-eight-week period. The first dose turned out badly, however, producing erosion. The dose was lowered, and Dr. Guthrie reports no incidence of problems with the lowered amount now used. He explained that the total amount, for the entire period, is less than that produced by the body in a single day and the use results in an extremely low incidence of contracture. "The implant is bathed locally in a fairly high concentration right around it, but not so high that it will get beyond the capsule."

He pointed out that the more amorphous the implant the better, because the less you're able to feel it and identify its edges, the more natural it is. Because the inflatable implants got off to several false starts, Dr. Guthrie feels that it will take another decade or so for them to be fully appreciated. Those surgeons who had bad experiences with them will never use them again, the way he will never use the polyurethane. They'd sooner take the problems with the others.

Dr. Guthrie has used all types in very large numbers (over one thousand of the saline-filled, over one thousand of the gel-filled, and about three hundred of the polyurethane) and feels that the saline is far and away the best. The silicone gel leaches out through the wall of the shell, so there are microscopic droplets of silicone found elsewhere in the body, each within its own capsule. He cited a recent report which revealed that women having silicone gel implants were found to have lymph nodes full of silicone. There were two reported cases of women having part of their lungs removed for coin lesions (round, coin-sized shadows on X ray) which were thought to be malignant but which were actually just siliconomas (localized collections of fibrous tissue stimulated by the presence of silicone). He feels that if the silicone's gotten as far as the lungs, it's certainly in the liver and kidneys.

He considers the double-lumen implant to embody the worst of both the gel and the saline. In those implants, he points out that the silicone leaches through two walls instead of one and there is still the possibility of leaking saline. He estimates that 60 to 90 percent of the double-lumen get hard as well. I asked why, then, do more than half the surgeons in the United States use gel-filled implants? His theory is that, unless a plastic surgeon is in a very large city or is known for a specific procedure, he performs the entire gamut of plastic surgery. Therefore, most plastic surgeons are not doing breast reconstruction in a very concentrated way. They may be told at a meeting that gel-filled implants are problematic, but that procedure accounts for only a very small percentage of their practice. He believes that if that was all they were doing, they would pay more attention to the report. Because of this, the ASPRS (American Society of Plastic and Reconstructive Surgeons) will not distinguish between the implants. They are all lumped together in one category, and Guthrie is afraid that the FDA will withdraw the inflatables as well as the gel-filled implants from the market.

In discussing appropriate implant size, he told me that the inflatable implants come in several standard sizes, from 125 cubic centimeters (cc) to 350 cc in 50 cc increments, the variety of sizes depending on the manufacturer. For instance, some companies will produce a 300 and a 350, while another a 275 and a 325. Standard sizes stop at around 300, 325, or 350, also depending on the firm producing them. That is only a large B cup or a small C cup, at the most. All manufacturers will make special-order implants as small as 90 cc and up to about a 600 cc, but there is a six-to-twelve-week wait on special orders. Dr. Guthrie therefore stocks them in 50 cc increments all the way up to 600 cc. He also keeps some 90 cc implants for augmentation of a very tiny breast on the other side in order to create a match. In terms of capacity, an implant can be filled to a little less than capacity or a little more (about 25 cc in either direction). If the level goes too far above, the implant gets too tight and feels hard; too far below, it gets too lax and wrinkles. Dr. Guthrie is prepared to use the very large implants to avoid surgery on the opposite breast wherever possible.

There is also a custom-fitted, gel-filled implant called the Birnbaum implant. It is made to order from a mold of the chest wall and resembles an external prosthesis. This is intended to fill out the sunken appearance created, in some cases, under the arm or the upper chest. In most instances, though, the standard range of implants will be satisfactory, and where the muscle is missing, the flap transplants will fill out the upper chest defect.

I had heard of "expanders," temporary implants used to gently stretch tight skin until a permanent implant can be inserted a few months later. There are two types; one is filled, through a tube, with saline over a period of weeks, and the other is filled with a concentrated salt solution, enabling it to soak up water on its own, by osmosis. The salt solution must be carefully worked out to determine the size when full. I asked Dr. Guthrie if he employed expanders. He replied that, in his view, there is a problem that renders them useless or dangerous. His explanation was that when the implant pocket is created, it is made very large, going well out to the side, well up, and right to the middle, so that the tissue can be stretched uniformly over a long distance. The expander is then inserted, and the tissue heals shut, so the only part of it being expanded is that right over the expander itself. That means that a small amount of tissue is being stretched a lot.

This puts enormous pressure on the skin and thins it out. The result is very thin fragile skin. He told me that it is also a little painful to be expanded and the final result is not very good. He would rather put in the largest implant possible for a patient and then change it in three months after the skin has stretched.

For women wanting to reconstruct the nipple-areola complex, Dr. Guthrie and most other plastic surgeons wait until three months after the creation of the breast mound. There are two reasons for this interim period. One is that when the implant is first inserted, it interferes with the blood supply. The blood has to come in from the sides instead of directly from behind; it's also being squeezed along its path of travel, so the blood flow over the central implant area is diminished. As Dr. Guthrie says, "That's not a good time to be planting a tree. It might not take." The second reason is that the breast changes its shape significantly in the first three months, and a nipple put on before then has a good chance of not being in the right spot later on. If that happens, you're stuck with it. Nipple-areola grafts can now be done on an outpatient basis under local anesthesia. You can be back home in two to three hours. Dr. Guthrie's favorite donor site for the nipple graft is from the labia majora, well away from the urethra and the vagina, almost in the groin crease. He likes the contrast color there. For the areola, he feels the ideal place is from the areola on the opposite breast, but that does leave a circular scar on that side which can be painful and visible and can interfere with sensation. So, unless he is doing another procedure on the other breast already, he doesn't use it. The next best place is the inner thigh, right next to the nipple site, but on the other side of the groin crease. Dr. Guthrie takes the nipple from one side and the areola from the other so that they won't pull against each other while healing.

The nylon stitches from the nipple-areola donor sites are left in for ten to fourteen days and the area remains tender during that period. Healing can be more uncomfortable in hot weather. At one point, Dexon self-absorbing sutures were tried, but the discomfort proved to be greater. As soon as the stitches are removed, patients report a rapid lessening of discomfort. Any scarring essentially disappears into the groin crease. The skin is naturally darker there, so it provides a contrast. It may look the same as the chest skin, but if you held your thigh up to your chest or your face (don't try it), you could see the difference. With my own areola graft site, although the scar is almost invisible (in the area over my appendix), fading occurred, and today it is considerably lighter than natural. When I mentioned the fact that other surgeons' favorite donor sites include earlobes and toes, Dr. Guthrie said that, in his experience, they tend to turn pasty-white.

I asked Dr. Guthrie about factors limiting reconstruction. He does not consider age a drawback, only health. He has recently reconstructed the breast of an eighty-seven-year-old who was highly motivated and delighted with the results. He said that although he wouldn't do a complicated procedure on someone that age, a straightforward implant insertion can be done on almost anyone, using a very light anesthetic.

I then asked whether radiation had any bad effects on the skin that might interfere with reconstruction. Dr. Guthrie explained that it causes irritation and swelling of the inner lining of the blood vessels. That blocks off the smaller vessels, which then clot and disappear. New ones come in, but they are not as good as the originals because the access of blood to the small vessels has been impeded. He said that the damage done to women by radiation varies considerably, but if the skin is brown-pigmented and leathery, the patient is not a candidate for reconstruction.

He went on to say that, even though chemotherapy slows down the healing process by interfering with cell production, some women on chemotherapy for two years are so unhappy about not having reconstruction that he does it for them. The only allowance he makes to the drugs is that he leaves the stitches in for ten days instead of six. He does not, however, do the nipple-areola grafts until after chemotherapy because the healing process is slow and a graft needs blood supply as quickly as possible in order to "take."

Dr. Guthrie does not do simultaneous mastectomy-reconstruction because he ran into the problem of the implants erupting through the incision. Instead, he prefers to wait a minimum of three months for the mastectomy scar to heal solidly and any inflammation or swelling to go out of the tissues. If, at three months postmastectomy, the skin is still tight, he waits three more months. The tissues do not stretch any more after six months, and that is when he makes his final judgment about the appropriate reconstructive technique. His advice to surgeons would be: "If you can't handle a patient with the procedures I've recommended, and you should be able to handle almost everyone, then don't do it."

One plastic surgeon specializing in using transplanted tissue and muscle without the need for an implant is Dr. Norman Hugo of Columbia-Presbyterian Medical Center, an affable bear of a man with an accent that brings to mind New England whaling towns and maple sugar. With energy and enthusiasm, he spoke about a new form of breast reconstruction, the RAM, otherwise known as the rectus abdominis myodermal flap. (Now you can see why it has a nickname.) This is a combination breast reconstruction and "tummy tuck" procedure. Although Dr. Hugo performs the more established methods of breast reconstruction, he has been devoting a great deal of his time to refining this new technique.

We spent the first part of my visit discussing the current "state of the art" of breast reconstruction. He, like many surgeons interviewed, commented that more younger women are coming in with breast cancer, women who will be physically and sexually active for many more years in the future. These women are demanding reconstruction and educating themselves to it. Patient age is not a consideration, he feels, but the state of health is. He believes that the woman is a better judge of her vitality than the surgeon, but if a patient, knowing that she has widespread disease, still wants reconstruction, he will not do it, because he feels that she is emotionally unable to make that decision.

He listed contraindications for breast reconstruction as inflammatory carcinoma (characterized by severe inflammation of the breast area); a big, fixed tumor limiting movement of the breast, which would presage an extremely high rate of disease recurrence; and multiple lymph node involvement. He does not believe that reconstruction causes recurrence of disease, but the cancer cells could possibly have been left there after the surgery. If there is a local recurrence, it is not deep but superficial, and therefore easily detectable. For delayed RAM surgery (not simultaneous with mastectomy), he requires that women be cancer-free for five years. Dr. Hugo emphasized that the patient must decide if the risk of the operation is compatible with her needs. She is the final judge of whether the result is worth the effort, particularly with the more complex procedures.

We began our discussion with the simpler breast reconstruction and then moved on to the more complex. With implant insertion, Dr. Hugo favors using the mastectomy incision rather than creating a new scar. When I asked why reconstructed breasts were rounder than the teardrop shape of the natural breast, he explained that, even if the prosthesis were shaped that way, the skin envelope keeps it from assuming a more relaxed shape. He told me that with very small breasts he usually doesn't do cosmetic work on the opposite side, and that the expander, which he puts right under the skin or behind the muscle, is good for small-breasted people with tight skin. Later on, he exchanges it for a silicone gel implant. However, he prefers the results obtained with the RAM procedure.

We moved on to the latissimus dorsi flap. This flap comes with a large amount of tissue, but it still doesn't provide as much tissue as the RAM. With the latter there is a very large block of tissue all living off one tiny little artery. Also, Dr. Hugo pointed out that all latissimus dorsi flaps require a silicone implant because there is not enough skin or tissue to make a breast mound. The RAM, however, brings enough of its own tissue to do so. With both of these procedures, the other breast can be "tucked" to match.

An advocate of simultaneous mastectomy and reconstruction, Dr. Hugo believes that healing is better and faster with that method than when reconstruction is delayed. His total operating time now is three and a half hours for the mastectomy and RAM reconstruction. With most surgeons doing this procedure (he estimates about ten in the United States), the time is about eight or nine hours. The recuperative period is also much lengthier than with a less complex procedure.

We visited the audiovisual department of the hospital to watch a videotape of a mastectomy and RAM procedure, which Dr. Hugo narrated. Before the tape started, he asked if this was the first operation I'd seen. I nodded, lips tightly sealed in the hope that I could avoid embarrassing myself all over the clean floor. To my surprise, after the initial incision, I felt perfectly fine. It all looked so neat, precise, and generally unmessy in contrast to what I had expected; a little like working on a machine. In fact, it was hard, after a while, to remember that that was a person up there.

In this technique, as the surgeon is performing the mastectomy, the plastic surgeon is separating a half-moon shape of the lower abdominal skin and fat from the surrounding structures on both hips. This shape is then picked up with the rectus muscle, which is the carrier and which comes with its own blood supply. One or both of the rectus muscles are picked up out of the abdomen and left attached to the half-moon of tissue. They are freed up all the way to the bottom part of the ribs. The skin is mostly stripped off the lower piece, except for a little island of skin to be used as in the latissimus dorsi. The rest of the muscle and tissue is fitted into the pocket in the chest. It eliminates the need for an implant and provides the skin for relaxation. A nipple is created, as early as one month later, by lifting out a plug of tissue to form a protrusion, which is more lifelike than the flatter grafts. This can be performed on an outpatient basis. I mentioned a brochure I had seen for a prosthetic, adhesive-backed nipple called the Knoche-Coury Nipple. The protrusion was very lifelike and the nipple, available in varying shades and sizes, was advertised as staying in place for up to six days at a time. Dr. Hugo told me that he uses such a prosthetic nipple to demonstrate to patients what the finished RAM nipple will be like.

With the RAM flap, both the natural droop and the softness of the breast are achieved. It is, after all, all your own tissue as opposed to an implant. However, it is much more difficult to judge the size of the breast, and Dr. Hugo acknowledges that the scarring is very apparent. There is also the risk of necrosis or death of the transplanted tissue. He points out that necrosis is very common among smokers (in fact, all of his necrotic patients were smokers) as well as among women suffering from decreased pulmonary (lung) function.

With removal of the abdominal support muscle, there is an increased danger of hernia. Dr. Hugo guards against this by flipping the fascia (a band of connective tissue) over the weakened area and securing it for support.

I interviewed several women who had undergone the RAM procedure within the past year, and although they were very pleased with the natural feel of the breast, they were concerned by the asymmetry. If the reconstructed breast is larger, however, that is easily correctable. Mostly, they were troubled by a thickened waistline and persistent stomach bulge.

Several surgeons interviewed expressed doubts about the RAM surgery. Dr. Guthrie was the most outspoken; he considers it an unacceptable procedure and provided a short anatomy lesson as background: "About halfway from the umbilicus to the pubic bone, the anatomy of the abdomen changes drastically. Above that point (called the semicircular line of Douglas), there are major supporting structures for the abdominal content behind the rectus muscle. Below that line, they are all in front of it.

"When you lift the rectus muscle, you have to lift all the

structures right in front of it because, if you didn't, you would disconnect the rectus from its overlying skin and fat, interrupting the blood supply between the two. There is nothing left between you and the peritoneal sac, which is paper-thin. Most important, the incidence of major lower midline abdominal hernia reported by the promoters of this operation is 10 percent in less than one year, and hernias only increase in number over a period of time. . . .

"The orthopedic community firmly believes that the two or three million people developing lower back pain in this country are getting it because of our docile way of life. We do not have the proper balance between the muscles in front and in back of the spine. Every one of these people is advised to strengthen the muscles in front. After the RAM, you cannot even do a sit-up because the principal muscle of the anterior [forward] abdomen has been removed." Many doctors fear that half of these women will develop chronic intractable lower back pain five to ten years after this surgery.

In rare cases, when a patient has had a very low mastectomy wound or a draining infection at the bottom of where the breast used to be, the rectus muscle can be safely flipped over, with skin on top of it. In that case, the section of muscle taken is from above the semicircular line of Douglas, which is much safer. The skin "island" won't die because it is all on top of the muscle, and since only some of the muscle is taken, it is still possible to do back-strengthening exercises.

In the RAM procedure, if the breast ends up too small or in the wrong position, you have to accept it, whereas, with implants, those changes can often be effected under local anesthesia. There are many women, though, who are more than willing to undergo this complex surgery to avoid having a foreign object in their bodies. The breast feels, they tell me, just like the natural one.

Dr. William W. Shaw is a microsurgeon at New York University Medical Center. At the end of a busy work day, we talked about his work with reconstructive breast surgery. He gives the impression of fastidiousness, and I could imagine him working for hours, meticulously reattaching tiny veins and arteries. We sat in his private ground-floor office, a garden visible through the large windows, the smiling faces of his young son and daughter in framed photographs on the bookshelves next to his desk. Dr. Shaw is soft-spoken, with an air of quiet elegance and a gentle manner. He was impressive in his attention to the whole woman, as involved with his patient's psyche as with her physical needs.

Although he performs the full range of reconstructive procedures, Dr. Shaw is responsible for the development of a procedure known as the superior gluteal microvascular free flap, known as the gluteal flap, which accomplishes breast reconstruction without silicone implants. He has been perfecting this process, first developed by Dr. Toyomi Fujino and reported in 1976, for five years. Up until one year ago, Dr. Shaw was the only one doing it in this country; now, he told me, there are perhaps one or two other surgeons employing the method. He said that five years ago a woman came to see him for breast reconstruction who was firmly opposed to an implant and did not want scarring on her upper back or abdomen. He modified Fujino's procedure and took the gluteal flap from the topside of one buttock, creating an implant-free reconstruction and leaving a scar that could be hidden by shorts or a bathing suit.

Dr. Shaw feels that the ideal method of reconstruction should satisfy the following criteria:

1. Simple in concept.
2. Limited and defined operations over a short time interval.
3. Permanency.
4. Ability to achieve aesthetic restoration of the skin surface, breast contour, and softness.
5. Minimal donor site disfigurement or function loss.

He began our interview with the statement that, with all the talk about breast reconstruction, some basic commonsense issues are not addressed. One is the emotional aspect. He thinks the view of breast reconstruction is positive, but that the whole concept of mastectomy and reconstruction implies two major emotional insults. The first is a true insult, while the second is an emotional change, albeit in a positive way. At times it can be negative because of expectations not fulfilled by surgery. He also believes very strongly in the different options. What upsets him is that the system seems to be more committed to competition between different methods. To start with, the anatomy is different for each patient, and so, therefore, are her requirements. For instance, he recommends silicone implants for two basic types of women. One would be the young mother with no nearby relatives to help out and an active schedule that would not permit time for a lengthy recuperation. The other type would be the older patient who is not as concerned with the cosmetic result as she is with replacing the breast mound. She doesn't want to spend a great deal of time recuperating, and her expectations are limited.

Dr. Shaw feels that many surgeons discuss reconstruction as an anatomic exercise when it should be tailored to the psychological needs as well as the physical ones. He hopes that the most important benefit is that reconstruction will enable women to come forth earlier in cases of suspected cancer, and emphasized that, the earlier the detection, no matter what method of surgery is employed, the better-looking the reconstruction. The field has improved enormously over the last ten years in terms of techniques and choices, and the woman, Dr. Shaw says, must know that there are options for her. He has seen many women, however, who are reluctant to take the responsibility of that choice. Options can make them nervous, but they may regret not taking a more active part in the decision later. Each patient is approached differently to work out the right surgery for her, the most important factor in reconstruction. Her feelings, personality, life situation, etc., must be considered.

Dr. Shaw pointed out that the term "breast reconstruction" is really a misnomer. "You can never really make a breast again. You try to restore the psychology and the feeling that the woman had preoperatively. The procedure should be termed a 'symbolic' reconstruction, since it is, after all, not her original breast being replaced." Dr. Shaw describes the ideal gluteal flap patient as young, wanting the best cosmetic result, having the time for it, and not wanting to incur the documented abdominal problems with the RAM. He states that some patients have described the silicone implant as "foreign" and always feel ill at ease with it.

Since the gluteal flap is a lengthy operation, age is a limiting factor. Dr. Shaw considers women up to sixty or sixty-five eligible. He reports that he does not see many women above that age interested in reconstruction anyway. He is emphatic that women should not be pushed into reconstruction; they should just be informed that they have the choice. A woman, he feels, can sometimes be pressured by lay articles or surgeons and may feel guilty that she is not seeking reconstruction. However, a woman pressured in this way is not a good candidate. There are times when he would suggest the gluteal procedure on an anatomical basis but the woman's personality is not suitable to difficult surgery. He tells the patient that, despite what he recommends, this must be her personal decision and that there is nothing wrong with doing something simpler or choosing not to reconstruct. Another point made was that some women love their buttocks more than their abdomens, and vice versa.

Dr. Shaw feels deeply the responsibility of presenting his suggestions to women, the risk being that they may be unhappy with the results. Most women, however, appreciate the time and explanation. They know that the final decision is theirs, and they are willing to accept that responsibility. If they can't make up their mind immediately, he encourages them to think about it and come back a second time to talk it over. "The woman must make the decision herself because the surgeon cannot assume the full responsibility for her happiness in any area of her life. She may say one thing to him, but what she really feels might be something very different. She may have personal reasons for making her final decision that she doesn't reveal to the doctor, but he feels better having presented the options thoroughly so she can make the ultimate move. The surgeon and the patient should be equal partners in the surgical process. The patient has to first come to terms with the disease and then try to pull herself together to make the most of her own life. Reconstruction is part of that second process."

Technically, Dr. Shaw says, it is possible to do the gluteal reconstruction simultaneously with mastectomy; in one way this is even easier, because the blood vessels are already accessible. But it would presently be a very long procedure. The operation is sound but very technical. It can be performed in about five or six hours, but, added to the mastectomy, that represents a long time on the operating table. It is technically possible, at this point, for him to do the procedure in four hours, but he acknowledges that it requires a very good microvascular surgeon. He commented that, once they see it performed, other surgeons can learn to do it quite easily. It is, however, extremely meticulous work. He worked on it for three years before even publishing a paper on it. He isn't aggressive in encouraging the procedure because a lot of women will request it and not every surgeon can do it well. "I'd rather work on it slowly, and as time goes on and the procedure becomes more and more organized, it will become a better operation for surgeons to handle."

Unlike the RAM surgery, in the gluteal reconstruction the artery is severed completely and the flap is moved to the chest and reattached, restoring the normal blood supply. This must be done fastidiously, since repair problems can result, causing the arteries to clot. The patient would then have to be taken back for surgical repair. Normally, patients are ambulatory about four days postsurgery. Dr. Shaw points out that the gluteal flap is a clean-cut piece, doesn't subtract anything vital, and achieves a much better result than the RAM flap. The artery and vein combination is tricky and tedious, but he is confident that he makes it work very well. The incidence of flap morbidity is much less than the abdominal flap, in Dr. Shaw's experience. Cosmetically, the breast reconstruction with the gluteal flap has a soft, natural bounce and the skin surface is soft and smooth. The donor site is left with a scar and an indentation that is not apparent in brief clothing. Dr. Shaw reports that patients do not seem to be bothered by that, much less than if it were a bulge in the lower abdomen. "That area of the buttocks is not prominent in the conscious mind anyway." The patients are more concerned with the lower part and are not able to see the donor site that easily themselves. Nipple-areola grafting is done two to four months later. Dr. Shaw states that, with the gluteal flap reconstruction, "the softness, projection, natural appearance, and patient satisfaction are excellent compared with other methods . . . the buttock area is also less painful for recuperation than the abdomen. With a young, active patient, this is the best reconstruction I can offer."

He considers the RAM technique a reasonable reconstruction without having to use an implant, but he always advises women of the complications. Coming back again and again with problems is psychologically debilitating for a woman. Also, he is wary of the eventual problems with the RAM, but he is still part of the group experimenting with such new techniques. He fears that there is a tendency in surgical reporting to emphasize the immediate positive aspects of a procedure without noting the long-term problems. Common complications of RAM surgery are necrosis, hernias, and the "belly bulge." Dr. Shaw says that the last one can be avoided, but it takes a great deal of time to dissect and close the fascia very, very carefully. It's not easy to do, and effecting a flat result is very painstaking. There is not much fat in most abdomens, even though women think there is, so it is hard to get a full breast.

I asked him to explain the basic differences between the gluteus and RAM procedures. "The RAM is not a free flap because it is left attached to the muscle and is notorious for not being hardy." The reason for that, Dr. Shaw theorizes, may be that the skin taken in the RAM procedure may not normally be supplied by the artery with which it is moved but by one down below. So, even though the skin may survive on that tiny artery, blood getting to the flap has a very long way to travel. He is beginning to think of trying the free-flap technique with the RAM procedure and then reattaching the flap in the hopes of avoiding some of the complications. He would hope to spare some of the abdominal muscle, as well, to minimize back and hernia problems. The gluteus method involves taking one muscle instead of two, as in the RAM. His fear is that a young woman will become pregnant after the RAM operation and have serious problems with the pressure on the abdomen. The same problems can occur as a woman grows fatter or older. Also, his observation is that the RAM flap does not fill out the hollowness of the radically mastectomized upper chest as effectively as the gluteus or latissimus dorsi.

He does very few latissimus dorsi procedures now because the scar on the back is too unsightly and visible. It also tends to widen in time. The skin taken from the back is thicker and coarser than normal breast skin, resulting in a minor color and texture difference in the reconstructed breast.

In discussing other possibilities for using the body's natural tissue in reconstruction, Dr. Shaw said, "Technically, it's an elegant thing to do to take part of the contralateral [opposite] breast to use in reconstructing the mastectomized one. The concept is lovely, but there is too great a risk of disease in that other breast to take the chance, and the result is no better than with the gluteal flap. Also, you've then scarred both breasts."

Simple Implant Insertion

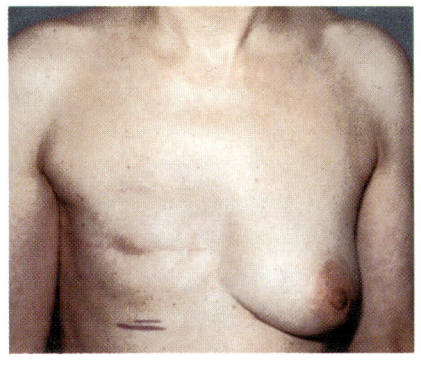

1. Post-mastectomy

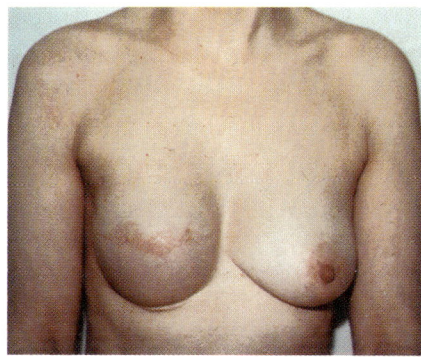

2. Implant insertion

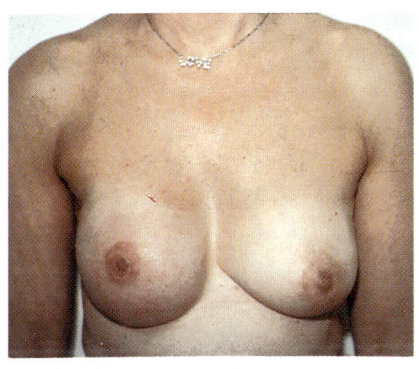

3. Nipple/areola grafts

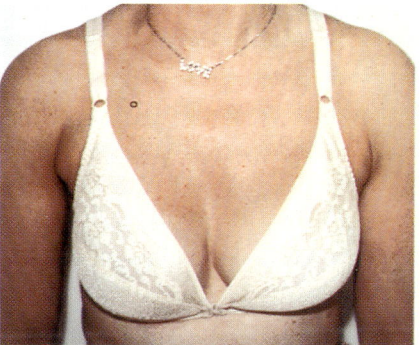

4. Reconstruction with bra

Simple Implant with Opposite Augmentation

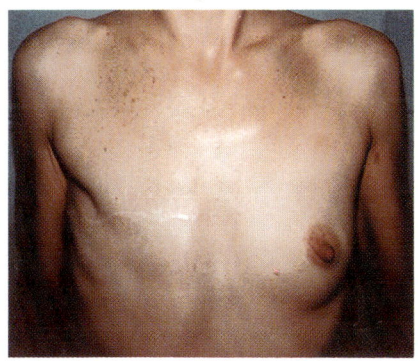

1. Post-mastectomy

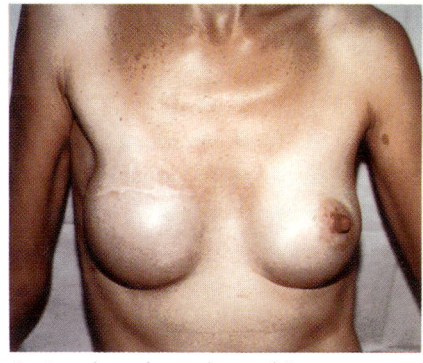

2. Implant insertion with opposite augmentation

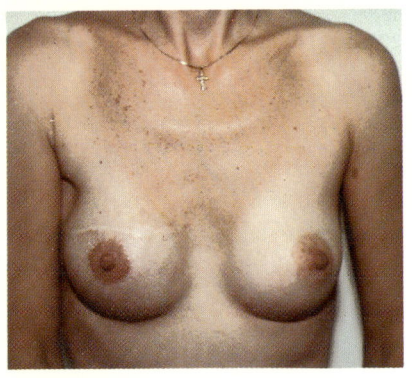

3. Nipple/areola grafts

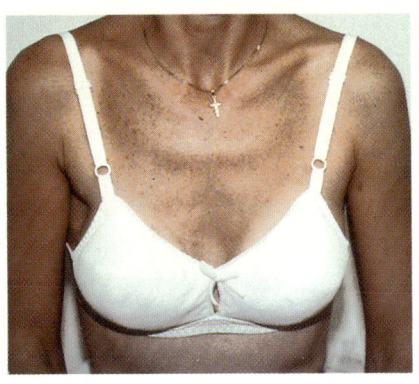

4. Reconstruction with bra

Simple Implant with Opposite Mastopexy

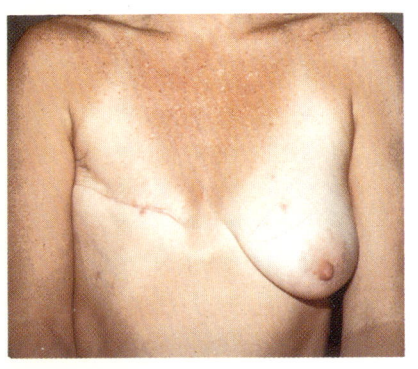

1. Post-mastectomy

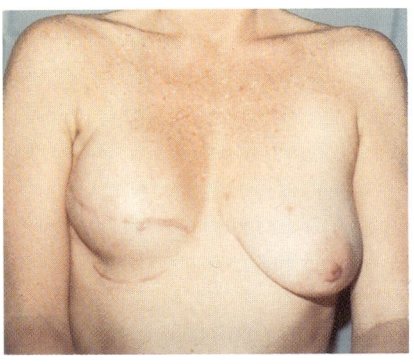

2. Implant insertion

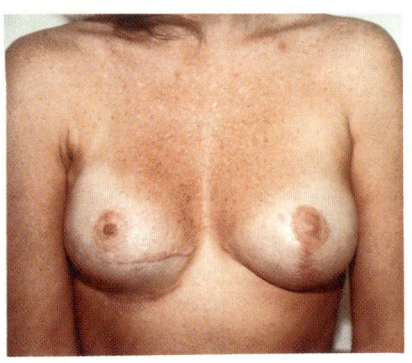

3. Opposite mastopexy and nipple/areola grafts

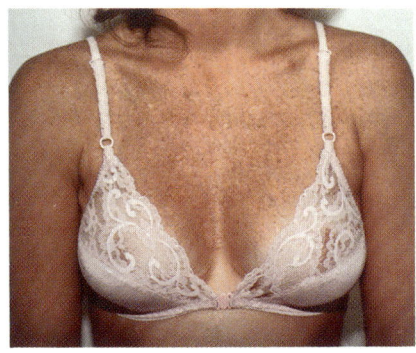

4. Reconstruction with bra

Latissimus Dorsi Flap

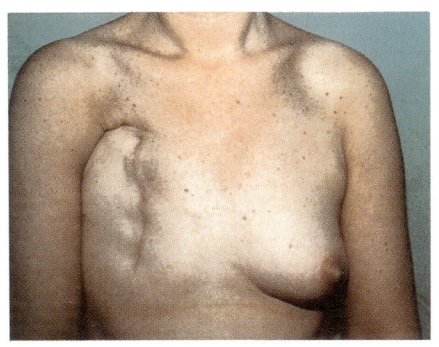

1. Post-mastectomy

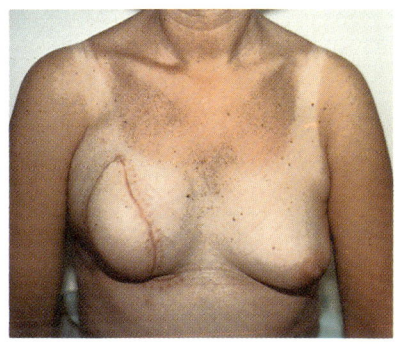

2. Latissimus dorsi

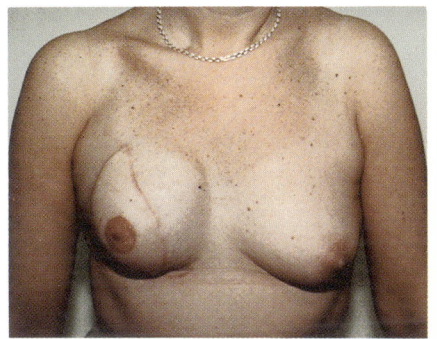

3. Nipple/areola grafts

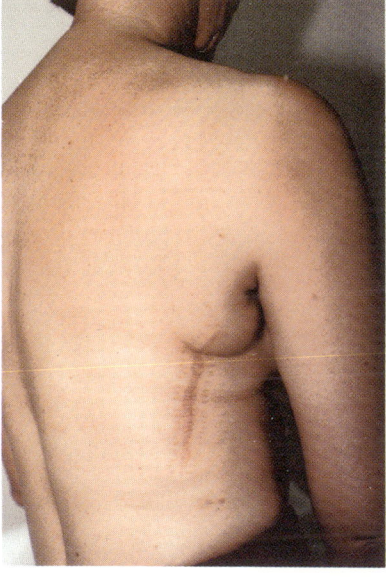

4. Donor site scar

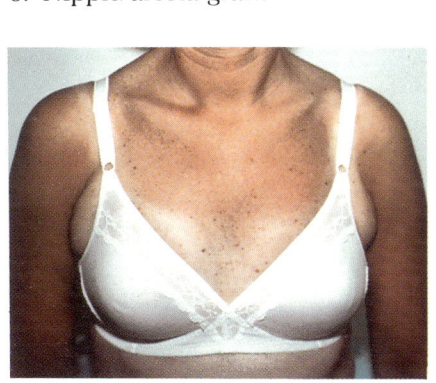

5. Reconstruction with bra

RAM Flap

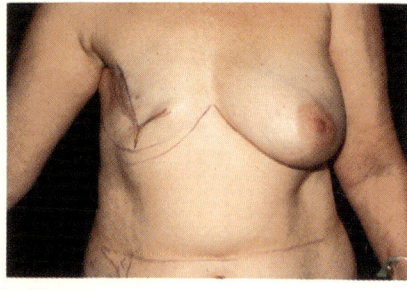

1. Post-mastectomy

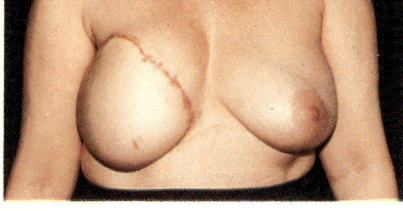

2. RAM

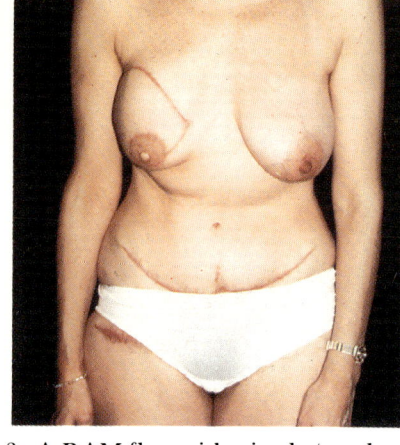

3. A RAM flap with nipple/areola grafts and donor site scar

Gluteus Flap

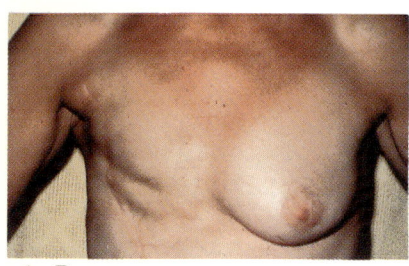

1. Post-mastectomy

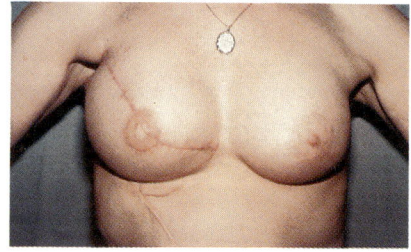

2. Gluteus flap, opposite augmentation, and nipple/areola grafts

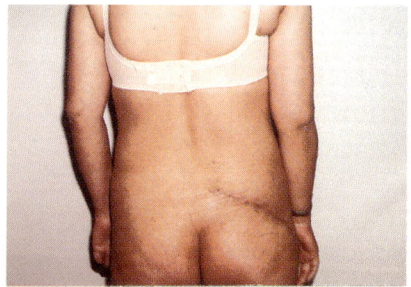

3. Donor site scar

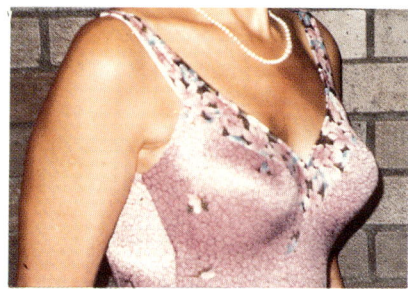

4. Reconstruction in bathing suit

When he does perform surgery on the other side for the purpose of achieving symmetry, Dr. Shaw reports that the incidence of sensitivity loss on that breast is not significant.

He expressed his worries about future problems with irradiated sites, in reconstruction and generally. He believes that, in five or ten years, we'll see a different generation of problems as the result of radiation. In terms of reconstruction, he feels that irradiated skin is not always problematic but that the surgeon does have to take it into consideration.

In terms of immediate versus delayed reconstruction, Dr. Shaw is of the opinion that it is not necessary for a woman to suffer a state of breastlessness before being rebuilt. He agrees, though, that this is a complex psychological issue that can be argued from both sides. In any case, he considers it inappropriate for the surgeon to say how a woman should feel. Women are highly variable in their reactions and must make that final decision themselves.

He related his most disappointing experience with breast reconstruction. It was after the best gluteal flap procedure he had ever performed on an ideal patient (young, positive, and anatomically well suited). He was puzzled to see her become depressed and difficult postoperatively when he had assumed that she would be thrilled with the results. "I was destroyed," he said. After talking with her, he found that she had, in spite of all cautions to the contrary, expected an exact replacement of her natural breast. As time went by, however, she told him that she was able to appreciate her new breast and derive much pleasure from it. Dr. Shaw, remembering, smiled with satisfaction.

I met with Dr. Saul Hoffman of Mount Sinai Hospital in New York City, a white-haired plastic surgeon with a ready smile, who was generous with his time and thorough in his explanations. He told me that he usually takes it for granted today that women do know about reconstruction and that their surgeons are discussing it with them, although he recognizes that there is still a big gap in the education. Women are demanding more information, and the American Cancer Society still seems unsure about how much they should get involved and what information to give out to the public. He is an adviser to the cancer society and is currently being consulted regarding their soon-to-be-released pamphlet on breast reconstruction, a companion to their slide presentation. Almost half of Dr. Hoffman's patients are breast reconstruction cases, even though he performs all types of plastic surgery.

I began by asking Dr. Hoffman where he prefers to make his incision for inserting an implant. He replied that he tries to go through the mastectomy wound in order to avoid creating another scar. If this wound is not in what he considers to be a good place, then he will create another opening. He said that he is now seeing more of the transverse (horizontal) incisions in mastectomy, rather than the oblique, and feels that the transverse is still the best. He observed that many surgeons don't use their imaginations; they don't vary the incision according to the location of the tumor or the chest configuration. Instead, they do what they're used to doing. If they consulted with a plastic surgeon, he feels, they might be able to choose another, better incision site. The cancer surgeons with whom Dr. Hoffman works are usually familiar with what he does and needs in terms of reconstruction. If there is a problem, they can talk with each other about it. That makes it more of a team effort. It helps a patient, too, if she consults a plastic surgeon before the cancer surgery so that she can view it as a collaborative effort, concerned not only with curing her but with rehabilitating her afterward. A woman will sometimes come to Dr. Hoffman with her own fixed ideas about breast reconstruction, and even though he might have suggested an alternative procedure, if he thinks her plan will work for her and she wants it badly, he goes along with it.

Dr. Hoffman favors the double-lumen implant. He had used the saline implants, which were softer than those containing silicone gel, but he had an entire series that leaked. He then decided that they weren't worth the headache for him or the trauma for the patients. He has been using the double-lumen for five years to "hedge the bet" but isn't sure yet if the results are really superior. He thinks, however, that the saline implants remain softer when they don't leak and they are also less likely to contract. He encourages his patients to massage their implants in an effort to avoid capsular contracture, explaining that the capsule sometimes shrinks down around the implant, squeezing it so that it feels hard. If a space can be maintained around and slightly larger than the implant, then there will be no pressure on it. By massaging it, moving it around, you can keep the capsule stretched out and tend to prevent its contracture. It doesn't always work, but it's one attempt to avoid the problem.

I asked Dr. Hoffman if he ever employs steroids to avoid contracture. He replied, "There is no doubt that it helps to prevent contracture but it is very difficult to control. There have been many complications from the use of steroids in implants. If there is too much, you'll have no formation of scar tissue and the implant will have no support. It can drop, or the skin over it can thin out." He will use steroids if a patient has had several procedures for repeated contractures, but he has to be very fastidious about the amount.

The nipple grafting is done three months postreconstruction on an outpatient basis. Dr. Hoffman uses the skin from the upper inner thigh, the opposite nipple, or the earlobe. The labia, he finds, is usually too dark, but he will use it for black women or white women with a very dark areola. The inner-thigh graft leaves a scar, but it is high up and doesn't seem to bother his patients. He also reports that the loss of sensation with reduction or lifting of the opposite breast is usually not a problem, although he prepares the patient for that possibility.

Dr. Hoffman began using expanders this past year for women with tight, thin skin. When he first started doing reconstructions, however, he used an inflatable implant intended as an expander. Saline solution was put into it with the idea of going back in and putting in more at subsequent operations. He found, though, that he could usually get enough volume in the implant during the first procedure. With very tight skin, however, he still had to expand it in stages, even though the idea of several procedures was not ideal. The point of the Radovan Expander, the one used now, is that it is meant to be expanded while in the patient, using a one-way valve right under the skin surface. Saline solution is injected through that valve over a period of time. Then the expander is removed and the implant inserted. The larger the pocket, the larger the prosthesis, but tight skin cannot be stretched all at one time. It is the same principle as if a pregnancy were a rapid, rather than a gradual, growth. It would tear the skin. The stretching of the breast skin is accomplished over a few weeks and is needed only in certain cases where the skin is too tight for an appropriate-sized implant. The expander is usually filled in one-week increments, and if there is any sensitivity in the valve area, a local anesthetic is used. Dr. Hoffman observed that since the expander is sometimes deliberately overexpanded for maximum skin stretching, it can look a little bizarre temporarily, but the final results of expanded patients are the same as with any good implant.

With reference to immediate reconstruction, Dr. Hoffman's reaction was "It has a place. The psychological benefits are certainly worthwhile, but I'm not sure that it should be done in every case. We do immediate reconstruction in cases where the tumor is noninfiltrating, but where we're not sure of the pathology report, we're not really pushing it. If the patient really wants it, we'll do it." He used to think that it was better to live with the mastectomy for a while, but has been shown that that is not true and that most women, if well prepared, are very happy with immediate reconstruction. On the "plus" side, also, it's easier to do the one-step procedure because everything is all prepared. There's no need to go back in again later. Dr. Hoffman feels, however, that there is slightly more incidence of complications, since, coupled with the mastectomy, it is a bigger operation. It can be a logistical problem for the plastic surgeon as well, since he would have to be available to do it at the time of mastectomy. If the surgeon has to order an implant in advance, he can't always judge, premastectomy, and may find, after all, that he doesn't have the right size to do the immediate procedure.

Commenting on the gluteal free flap procedure, Dr. Hoffman said that, so far, Dr. Shaw is the only one he knows doing it. He feels that only someone like Dr. Shaw, an extremely accomplished microvascular surgeon, can do it. He has seen some of Dr. Shaw's work and is highly complimentary. He said that the gluteal flap may, in time, become the standard operation, but it is not done that commonly now because of length, lack of skilled surgeons, and potential complications. Dr. Hoffman has, however, referred patients to Dr. Shaw when he felt that none of the other procedures were going to be satisfactory for them. There is a tendency with new procedures, he cautioned, to want to do them to everybody, and sometimes that can be a mistake. "It [the gluteal free flap] has a very prominent place in the gamut of what we can offer patients, but it's certainly not at the top of the list at this point."

Dr. Francis Symonds of Columbia-Presbyterian Medical Center is an elegant, silver-haired plastic surgeon, gentle and thoughtful in manner. We met in his office in a large building housing scores of identical medical suites. Even the waiting rooms on each floor are exactly alike. We began by discussing some surgeons' fear that reconstruction would mask a recurrence of disease. Dr. Symonds pointed out that the incidence of cancer recurrence in the chest wall is relatively small and the likelihood of curing it, if it does recur there, is very low. Therefore, the patient would not have an advantage in that case without the implant. On the other hand, an implant pushes the soft tissue forward, facilitating self-examination and detection of recurrence in that area.

Dr. Symonds feels that, as the public becomes better informed, more women will demand reconstruction. The problem now is that not very many are even aware of the option.

He has also performed immediate reconstruction and reports that it is becoming much more common, negating the need for a woman to go through that awful period of breastlessness. "When we first started, we thought that if we couldn't come up with something that was exactly like her natural breast, then it was better for her to be with no breast for a while so that, when we replaced it with something, she wouldn't be so disappointed. But now the technique has improved to the point where some immediate reconstructions are so good that we don't feel that way."

On the subject of tight capsules, Dr. Symonds says that it is impossible to tell why one woman's body will develop that complication while another's will not. A capsule will always form around any foreign body, but some contract and others don't. He is emphatic, however, that the release of steroids from the implant to avoid contracture is not an accepted procedure because of their potential danger. He acknowledges that even though the silicone in the gel-filled implants can be demonstrated as migrating throughout the body, there is no evidence that there is any harm in that at all.

Dr. Symonds's opinion concerning the RAM procedure is that it works best in the woman who is a little heavy, has had two or three children, and has loose abdominal skin. I asked what could be done for the woman who had undergone a quadrantectomy, which removed approximately one quarter of the breast, leaving a considerable defect. He described restoring the missing area by using a tiny implant and adding grafted skin.

In a "matching" procedure on the other breast, if there is loss of sensitivity, Dr. Symonds explained that it is in the lower part of the breast and that there is also complete or partial loss of nipple-areola sensation. Insurance companies, in his experience, are more likely to cover surgery on the opposite breast if it is done at the same time as the reconstruction on the mastectomized breast.

Dr. Mary McGrath of Columbia-Presbyterian Medical Center is a young plastic surgeon specializing in immediate breast reconstruction. She has a brisk, efficient manner and a *very* firm handshake. I first heard her speak about her work at the New York University Breast Cancer Symposium and later met with her in her hospital office. Clear in her explanations and determined in style, she brought to mind my nononsense ninth grade grammar teacher, Miss Marsh. She was demanding, but it was worth it.

Dr. McGrath has recently completed a study comparing the physical and psychological effects of immediate versus delayed reconstruction, done in cooperation with a psychiatrist, Dr. Laurie Stevens. This was prompted by the current concern among patients and surgeons being not so much whether to reconstruct a breast but when. She began her report by listing three major concerns in making the decision: the psychological impact of the timing, the medical safety, and the technical considerations on the part of the reconstructive surgeon. She addressed the point made by critics of immediate reconstruction that it was wiser to wait until the highest risk for local recurrence of disease has passed, quoting recent studies that indicate that the period between mastectomy and local recurrence is much longer than the two years previously used as a guideline. The most important indication of local recurrence is still the degree of lymph node involvement at the time of the mastectomy. Dr. McGrath listed the results of a study done at the M. D. Anderson Clinic in Houston, Texas: "For Stage I patients, a mean of 6.2 years elapsed before local recurrence. None recurred before two years. For Stage II, it was 4.2 years, and for Stage III, an average of 2.1 years." She pointed out that a large majority of local recurrences were in the mastectomy scar, making them readily detectable even with reconstruction. Dr. McGrath concludes, "For the Stage I patient, the risk is no greater with immediate reconstruction than with a procedure that's being delayed several months or a few years."

When I asked Dr. Robert Somers for his views on immediate reconstruction, he said he formerly opted for delayed reconstruction because he felt that an immediate procedure enabled the patient to deny the cancer to a dangerous degree. He now recognizes the psychological benefits of immediate reconstruction, and if his immune surveillance theory is correct, that may be a good argument for immediate reconstruction, thereby eliminating the need for a separate surgical procedure.

In the McGrath/Stevens study, the candidates for immediate reconstruction were told that if, in the operating room, the frozen-section examination of the lymph nodes indicated disease spread, then reconstructive surgery would not be done at that time. Although none of the women had any evidence of spread on frozen section, the subsequent laboratory pathology yielded microscopic nodal involvement in five out of thirteen instances. Reconstruction was done using a latissimus dorsi flap with an implant or with a submuscular implant alone. The decision on the procedure was made with the patient before the surgery, according to her body contour and the opposite breast. Women requiring chemotherapy began their treatment after the usual mastectomy wound-healing period. Their course of therapy was not altered in any way by the reconstruction or the prosthesis, nor was there any incidence of implant infection. Dr. McGrath emphasized that "a properly planned and executed reconstruction, with or without a myocutaneous flap [a flap consisting of skin and muscle], would heal as consistently and as rapidly as a mastectomy wound. Infection is relatively uncommon with the use of mammary prostheses. About 70,000 implanted devices are used yearly in this country, approximately one third of them for breast reconstruction, and the overall incidence of infection is less than 1 percent of cases. This may be due to the avascular [without blood supply] fibrous capsule that forms within two weeks around the silicone breast prosthesis, or it may be related to the submuscular placement of the prosthesis. There is now early experimental evidence that bacteria are cleared more rapidly beneath a well-vascularized, well-oxygenated muscle cover than beneath subcutaneous tissue or skin flaps."

Regarding the question of silicone implants absorbing radiation during radiotherapy, Dr. McGrath reported that "the prosthesis itself will tolerate up to 10,000 rads over four weeks without any change in physical characteristics." The maximum recommended radiation dosage for treatment is well below that figure.

Dr. McGrath acknowledged that not all the factors determining the choice of reconstructive procedure can be determined before the mastectomy. There is, for example, an unpredictable variation in the tightness and thickness of the breast flap. She agreed that this inhibits the general acceptance of immediate reconstruction, since "it requires either a highly consistent ablative surgeon [the one treating the disease] or a highly flexible reconstructive surgeon or maybe a little of both."

There is, according to proponents of immediate reconstruction, significantly less bleeding with immediate reconstruction than with delayed. Dr. McGrath explained that it is technically easier to deal with tissue that is fresh, not already scarred; the bleeding is more easily controlled.

I asked her about loss of sensitivity after surgery on the opposite breast. Roughly one third of her patients, she told me, report no change in sensitivity, one third a decrease, and one third an increase. For implants, she prefers the double-lumen and took one out of her desk drawer to show me. Plopped on the desk top, it looked like a sandwich-sized plastic bag filled with a clear gel and a liquid. She also told me that she does not do nipple reconstruction at the same time as the breast mound because, aesthetically, it is not acceptable. Instead, the nipple-areola complex is done three months later as an outpatient procedure.

Addressing the implant controversy, Dr. McGrath provided some background information: "In 1976 the Medical Devices Act was passed by Congress requiring that all implantable medical devices be classified as either 1, 2, or 3 and absolutely proven safe for patient use. Almost all other implantable devices are in Class 3. Breast implants came up for classification for the first time last year, and like most other implants, they're being put into Class 3. This means that there is a period of pre-market surveillance after which they may or may not pass and move into Class 2 or they will remain in Class 3. If something negative came up, they would be removed from the market. This is true of all medical devices. There has been a tremendous and unfortunate concern about this, and the erroneous implication is that they have been dropped from a better category. Actually, this will now give us an opportunity to separate breast prostheses into different groups. For instance, polyurethane prostheses should not be in the same category as the gel-filled or saline ones."

Dr. McGrath feels that a good deal of damage has been done to the field of breast reconstruction by articles written by a *Washington Post* reporter, Judith Randall, who considers breast augmentation an abrogation of women's rights and dignity. Her widespread stories, carried in publications as varied as *The New York Times* and the *National Enquirer*, accuse plastic surgeons of defining a small breast as a deformity and imposing male standards of breast appreciation on women. When confronted, Ms. Randall states that she is referring only to cosmetic breast enlargement, but, by association, the breast reconstruction field is suffering as well. Dr. McGrath is convinced that this is all part of the groundless fear being generated about breast prostheses in general.

In discussing the psychological repercussions of mastectomy, Dr. McGrath compared postmastectomy depression to that experienced in mourning the loss of a loved one. (My own reactions to my breast loss, exactly! It's always comforting to realize that those deep, dark feelings during hard times are shared by others; it helps one feel less isolated.) She reported that two and a half years ago she and Dr. Stevens began their study to determine whether this mourning process was altered in women undergoing simultaneous mastectomy and reconstruction. Dr. Stevens conducted in-depth psychological interviews of both groups of women. The women in the immediate group were found to have fewer symptoms of depression than those delaying reconstruction, and the latter group reported that their feelings of depression lessened after reconstruction. They had also expressed feelings of deformity, postmastectomy, but the immediate group had none. Almost all of the women undergoing immediate reconstruction said that they considered the surgery to be a restoring of the breast, whereas most of the delayed group referred to it as a replacement. The idea that the immediate reconstruction could enable a woman to forgo the incredibly painful adjustment to an altered body image negates a good deal of the emotional horror associated with breast cancer.

I then met with Dr. Stevens, who elaborated on the study's findings. I played the role of devil's advocate by raising the opposition's arguments against immediate reconstruction: (1) Postmastectomy women need a period of adjustment to the trauma and loss before rebuilding a breast; (2) immediate reconstruction fosters denial of the disease; and (3) without an interim period of breastlessness, the new breast will be unfavorably compared to the natural one.

Dr. Stevens responded that she had seen no convincing evidence, to date, which proves that you have to live with a mastectomy defect in order to be satisfied with a reconstruction. She reported that all but one of the women she studied were 100 percent satisfied with their breasts, whether they had immediate or delayed reconstruction. The one dissatisfied woman, in the immediate group, had a fantasy that she would have large breasts after the operation. She never shared those thoughts with her doctor prior to surgery, and if they had been known, she could have discussed the possibility of a larger reconstructed breast and an augmentation of the opposite normal breast. Dr. Stevens said, "One of the most important things we have learned from our study is to ask women about their fantasies and whether they have been happy with their breast size. Some feel that their breasts were too large and almost prefer the reconstructed breast to the natural one, calling it 'my adolescent breast' because it's small, firm, and doesn't sag. They will often have the other one reduced to accomplish body symmetry. That dispels the myth that women won't want to have any kind of cosmetic surgery on the remaining healthy breast."

On the question of acceptance of the natural breast loss with immediate reconstruction, Dr. Stevens observed that many of her immediate-reconstruction patients do feel appropriately sad about the loss but do not have the more devastating psychological reactions of the women who live with the mastectomy. She also emphasized that immediate reconstruction can offer restoration of the lost breast without the patient having to endure the extreme emotional trauma of being breastless. The immediate-reconstruction group integrated their new breast into their body image better than the delayed group. They feel that it is a real part of them rather than something foreign, stuck on their chest wall, and have fewer inhibitions about touching it than do the women delaying the reconstruction. Neither immediate nor delayed reconstruction enables a woman, however, to forget that she has had a serious disease. Overall, women who had immediate reconstruction experienced significantly less psychological trauma in many areas studied. They had a much lower incidence of depression and not as much lowering of self-esteem, their feelings of femininity remained intact, and they reported a more rapid return to sexual functioning. (From my own point of view, not having to deal with a prosthesis or change wardrobes would provide another "plus." I can remember angrily ripping all of the low-cut, revealing dresses out of the closet one day. How nice it would have been to avoid that outer change when I had to deal with so many inner changes.)

Dr. Stevens mentioned that the women in the immediate group on chemotherapy had much more difficulty in adjusting to the accompanying hair loss, chemically induced depression, and loss of libido than to the reconstruction. They would say, "The breast is fine. It's all this other stuff that's driving me crazy!"

She also reports that even when women without cancer have breast surgery, they can have enormous fears of body dissolution. With breast-reduction surgery, they sometimes have dreams and fantasies of their incisions opening, allowing all of their breast tissue to fall out. "The problems of operating on a part of the body that juts out into the world, like a breast or a leg, are much greater from a body-image point of view," says Dr. Stevens. "The patient can touch that part, whereas something like a gallbladder is inside and doesn't seem as real a loss. It's as if they have a zipper that is opened up when you operate and then zipped up again. The patient has a sense of mystery about what's in there." That issue becomes even more complex with the breast, which is a maternal organ as well. One woman who had previously decided not to have children had an overwhelming urge to have them after her reconstruction. Dr. Stevens feels that her new need was directly related to the sudden alteration of her breast and, after having cancer, her desire to produce something to carry on her legacy.

I know many mastectomized women who have come to terms with their breastless state and seem truly at peace, whereas others are still defensive on the subject of reconstruction. In studies done by Drs. Marcia and John Goin of the Departments of Psychiatry and Plastic Surgery at the University of Southern California School of Medicine, the phrase "pseudo-acceptance" was defined. Drs. Goin and Goin believe that some women go through loss, denial, anger, and depression before entering a stage of pseudo-acceptance. Others go through a genuine bargaining period that evolves into a real acceptance. The pseudo-acceptance, on the other hand, is a kind of resignation in which they will acknowledge that they have gone through a difficult time but, at a certain point, have come to feel fine about it. Underneath, this group of women is still very depressed and defective-feeling. The study concludes that it is these "pseudo-acceptors" who go on to seek delayed reconstruction and are very happy with the restoration of the lost body part. The reconstruction eventually causes them to become true acceptors.

Dr. Stevens has observed that women are equally concerned with the threat of cancer and the breast loss. At Columbia-Presbyterian Medical Center, where the McGrath/Stevens study was conducted, they found that it was extremely helpful if one member of the team on each breast cancer case was a woman. That is now their recommendation in all future treatment: a female surgeon and/or a female psychiatrist with whom the patient can discuss feelings. Women badly need one of their own as counsel. Many ask their doctors if anyone who has been through the experience is available to talk to them—a positive example, someone who's "been there." Ex-patients are very often evangelistic about their reconstructions because they feel it made such a positive difference in the quality of their lives.

In my own research into this topic, I found that surgeons who are sensitive and educated to the alternatives are now mentioning reconstruction as a possibility when they present the original surgical options. They also make decisions about when, in the course of treatment, the women should have reconstruction. At times surgeons assume that an older woman would not want or need it, so in those cases it often goes unmentioned. In Dr. Stevens's group, however, there was an immediate-reconstruction patient in her sixties with very little sexual involvement. In her case, reconstruction had to do with restoring her body integrity. The youngest patient in the study was twenty-eight, and there was a delayed reconstruction on a seventy-five-year-old. In a study of postmenopausal mastectomized women, Drs. Goin and Goin reported that "during frequent open-ended interviews, feelings were revealed of loss, depression, and shame about sexual feelings that they believed to be inappropriate to their age. The patients' need to pretend to themselves and others that the mastectomy was relatively unimportant added an extra burden to the usual stress of coping with midlife anxieties.

However, reconstruction decreased the mastectomized woman's feelings of dependence and mutilation."

In a recent article in *Sexual Medicine Today*, Dr. Bromley S. Freeman, Clinical Professor of Plastic Surgery at Baylor College of Medicine in Houston, Texas, writes that "to many women, mastectomy has implications similar to those of castration. 60% of the women surveyed in a recent Gallup poll said their womanhood would be impaired if they had to undergo a mastectomy. 18% felt the loss of a breast carried far more significance than the loss of a limb, and 9% said they would rather die." With 90,000 mastectomies performed yearly, this represents an overwhelming psychological threat to the lives of all women. A promise of reconstruction "can shorten the depression and aid the physical and social rehabilitation." He goes on to say: "Breast reconstruction promotes more positive attitudes about self, sexuality, and the quality of life. On the basis of these factors, it should be offered more widely. The mastectomy should be performed with reconstruction in mind; surgical incisions should be made in the least visible areas. Breast reconstruction should follow as soon as possible. Research indicates mammoplasty reduces anxiety about sexual arousal in mastectomized women. It also appears to reduce the feelings of loss (including grief and depression) and the anxiety about sexual functioning."

Dr. Freeman concludes that, regardless of the patient's age or how long ago she had a mastectomy, she should be provided with information about reconstruction. Surgeons using age as a negative for reconstruction are wrong to do so because it depends on the individual and her vitality, not on her years. I feel strongly that this is another negative result of living in a youth-oriented culture where anyone over a certain age is assumed to be lacking in life drive and sexuality.

I interviewed Dr. Ellen Jacobs, a clinical psychologist who, with Memorial Hospital's Dr. Jimmie Holland (Chief of the Department of Psychiatry) and Dr. Ted A. Chaglassian (Chief of the Plastic Surgery Service) participated in a three-year study funded by the National Cancer Institute on emotional response to breast reconstruction. Two groups were studied. The first group chose reconstruction and were followed from postmastectomy to at least three months postreconstruction. The second group of women did not choose reconstruction. The study was conducted from May 1980 through April 1983 and was a psychological and surgical evaluation. The women in the first group were found to be psychologically well adjusted to the reconstruction and very satisfied. The study, as yet unpublished, also addressed the difference in adjustment between postmastectomy and postreconstruction.

I spoke to Dr. Jacobs about her own reactions to the women studied. There was a small group, she reported, that was somewhat defensive about their decision not to undergo reconstruction. At that point in time, they were enough at peace with themselves and with how their lives were going to decide against it. It was hard to tell, she said, in a single interview with these women whether some form of denial was operating, but if it was, it was working well. It is hard to predict who will pursue reconstruction and who will not. One of the ways in which many women have coped with mastectomy has been to master it, to rise above it. Women who underwent mastectomy long before reconstruction was available are being told now that, if the timing had been different, they could have been spared suffering by undergoing reconstruction. Dr. Jacobs feels that the new option of reconstruction is disturbing to those women who thought they had made peace with the situation. Also, some women who would not consider reconstruction for years after mastectomy may go through a change in their lives such as divorce or career change and suddenly decide that they want to replace the missing breast.

Dr. Jacobs observed that the clinic patient who has had reconstruction is rare at this point. The "word" has not reached that segment of the population yet. There are many hospitals outside the major metropolitan areas where reconstruction is still not being mentioned even though breast cancer has reached epidemic proportions. Her final observation was that women who have had reconstruction could not wait to share it. One of the best things about doing the Memorial study, she said, was how willing the women were to participate when they felt they might be able to help someone else.

7

A Range of Experience: Monologues

This chapter needs no explanation; the voices of the following women, my "sisters," will suffice. I have changed names to ensure the privacy of their intimate revelations, but their stories illuminate the spectrum of the postmastectomy experience and subsequent rehabilitation. It does not matter whether or not they chose reconstruction as their route; they all traveled the road to recovery in their own time and manner.

One important point: when I began my interviews, I was determined to provide as broad a socioeconomic range of opinion as possible. Well, I was naïve to say the least. It was a cinch to find women in my own general category, living in major metropolitan areas, able to afford expert medical care, and with the time to do their own research and networking. It was quite another story when I attempted to unearth cases of clinic reconstruction. The more elusive these examples became, the more obsessive I became in my search. When I asked a plastic surgery resident in a major metropolitan teaching hospital why there are so few reconstructions among clinic patients, he replied, "Simple. The cancer surgeons do not refer the clinic mastectomy patients to us, and the patients don't know about reconstruction to ask for it. Also, Medicaid pays so little that the hospital loses money on the procedure."

Another hospital denied my requests to interview their clinic mastectomy patients, even though I promised anonymity for both hospital and patients, because they felt that "in the framework of their [the patients'] life situation, informing them of reconstruction could only make them feel worse than they already do."

Sue Lucas, my Reach to Recovery reconstruction contact in Mississippi, reports that she has great difficulty finding minority volunteers who have had reconstruction to do counseling work. She feels that the perception of cancer in those segments of society is still "You do not admit it, talk about it, or share your feelings." She recently sent out fifteen hundred invitations to clinic patients to attend a breast cancer forum, and only five or six attended. One clinic patient came forth to have reconstruction in the hope that her husband, who had deserted her after the mastectomy, would return. When Sue visited her in the hospital, she admitted that, even if he did not come back, she was thrilled that she had gone through with the surgery.

I asked several Hispanic acquaintances if they knew of reconstructed women in their communities. Without hesitation, their reply was that no one they ever knew had even had a mastectomy—a statistical improbability today. Even with the success stories associated with breast cancer, it is still treated, in many quarters, as the twentieth century's equivalent of leprosy or the plague, and the women who are least able to fend for themselves emotionally and financially are still those most isolated in their grief. One nursing supervisor told me of her frustrating struggle to convince many of her clinic patients to part with a badly diseased breast. In her view, "for a great many of these women, the breast *is* the woman. They would rather die than lose it." If the message about reconstruction is able to reach them, then perhaps more lives will be saved. It is my firm belief that, once informed, more clinic patients will demand their right to exercise that option. The medical community and health care system will yield to the societal pressure. But until then, as the supervisor said, "if you don't know about it, you can't ask for it."

JOAN

I had my mastectomy six years ago. When I was a kid, I was a tomboy and I developed late. I can remember being excited that I could finally wear a bra, and I liked the way my breasts looked. In sex, they weren't that important to me, though. [*Laughing.*] I liked other things.

The way I knew I had cancer was that I insisted on a two-stage procedure, and when I woke up after the biopsy, I knew I had a malignancy because of the way the stitching was done. I used to work in a hospital, so I could tell. After my mastectomy, I thought only about the disease. I wasn't that "attached" to the breast. I was more afraid of missing out on life. I was terrified of a slow death that would debilitate everybody around me. I knew I was a survivor because, two days after surgery, I dragged myself to the sink and washed and dried my hair with my one good arm while my roommate screamed that I was crazy. [*Laughs.*]

I have two teenaged children and my husband was extremely supportive during my illness. We discussed reconstruction early, but initially I was reluctant. My surgeon presented the option but advised me to wait for two years in case of a recurrence. While I was in the hospital, I did speak to a Reach to Recovery volunteer. She and the nurses helped me make the adjustment. One day, a couple of months later, my husband announced that he was leaving me and the kids. He denied that the breast was part of it, but, traditionally, he had a very tough time dealing with illness. I knew him well enough to know he couldn't take it. After he left, I went into therapy for a little while, but I didn't feel I needed it. I just wanted to make sure that it wasn't something I did that made him go.

Then one day, two years later, I was getting dressed for

work and I was putting on my bra with that heavy thing [the prosthesis] in it, and I said to myself, "This is dumb!" I went to work and asked a doctor at the hospital to recommend a plastic surgeon, which he was happy to do. I didn't go to see any other surgeons; I had faith in his referral. I wouldn't have known how to "shop around," anyway. Sometimes I wonder, though, if I should have. But after my husband left and all, I really felt like doing something for myself. I said to myself, "If I never do anything else, this is my gift to me, not for anybody else."

I consider the plastic surgeon an artist. He had to do a latissimus dorsi flap because I didn't have enough skin. I didn't expect that it would be just like the other breast since I had seen other reconstructed women at the hospital where I work. The first reconstructed woman I ever saw was a grandmother.

We did a two-stage procedure, and in the second stage the other breast was "tucked." The areola graft was from the upper inner thigh, and a vaginal graft was used for the nipple. The thigh scar is high up in the crease, and I grow two tiny pubic hairs on that areola now as a result. They don't bother me at all. I think I had three hairs on there before! The doctor likes to tweeze them when I go back for checkups. [*Laughs.*] I guess he doesn't like to see his artwork spoiled.

The reconstructed breast has dropped a little now and it's a little smaller than the natural one. I could go back to make the alterations, which would be minor, but I don't want to bother. On the other hand, the bilateral reconstructions that I've seen look perfect to me.

Emotionally, I'm elated! It's wonderful to look down and see cleavage again! And when my natural breast was tucked, there was no loss of sensation. My insurance paid for almost everything. I have Blue Cross/Blue Shield and Major Medical. I have a very supportive family and friends. I'm just grateful that I came out of this whole thing okay. The fact that I had all of these avenues and options open to me was wonderful, and reconstruction worked well for me. I hope other women will learn that they can have this, too. They'll feel reimbursed.

At work I use myself as an example for women interested in reconstruction. I work in X ray, and sometimes women come in who are reconstructed. Women should remember, by the way, to tell technicians about their implants before they have X rays or bone scans. It isn't harmful in any way, but they should know it's there. Some women are so miserable and angry when they're undergoing chemotherapy, they can't see past it. Others get excited at the thought of reconstruction. I offer to show them mine, and suddenly they can see beyond what they're going through at the moment. I haven't met one woman who is violently anti-reconstruction. Those who are negative about it are more afraid of surgery than anything else. Some women say to me, "How could I have caught cancer?" or "I come from a family of all men. We don't get this!" They desperately need a rationale and can't find it. I see no difference in attitude toward reconstruction based on background or income, but I feel that most poor women don't even know that it's available. I've even introduced women to each other at the hospital who have had or are interested in having reconstruction. One woman found fault with every plastic surgeon she interviewed, so I told her, "Forget it, you're just not ready." A woman has to be highly motivated to have reconstructive surgery, and it's got to be because she wants it, nobody else. I tell the women, "This has got to be the best thing you do after you've been through the pits. If you have to go through hurt, this is a hurt that's worth it."

LAURA

I had a radical mastectomy as a clinic patient over eleven years ago. I'm divorced now and I have two children. I have to tell you that I would still make that mastectomy choice today, as well as the one-stage procedure. Getting the disease out was paramount for me. The sense of isolation was the worst part of the whole experience. I have not had reconstruction. It was not available then, and I have thought of it since only in the abstract sense. I've learned to live with my body and it doesn't make me uncomfortable. Also, the surgeon did not, of course, do the mastectomy with reconstruction in mind at that time. I think it would be a very complex procedure in my case, if not impossible, but I don't even feel motivated to look into it. Besides, I don't want more surgery of any kind. I never want to see the inside of a hospital again, thank you very much! [*Laughs.*]

I'm a social worker now and I counsel many women pre- and postmastectomy. I really think that counseling prior to mastectomy is critical but still very inadequate; it's not available to enough women. Also, I think it's better if the counselors have had the mastectomy and reconstruction experience themselves. I was in therapy at the time of my illness, and I felt that the therapist had an analytical, rather than humanitarian, approach. She hadn't had a mastectomy. I needed someone who could say, "Hey, I've been there and I got through it. You can, too."

SUZANNE

When I was thirteen, I remember I wanted a bra because my breasts began to hurt. I loved the bra straps because the boys could feel them and they'd know I was a woman. I didn't think my breasts were perfect, though; I wanted tiny, uplifted ones. I've never felt good about my body, in general, but I always loved my breasts. I loved being a woman because of them and would fondle them when I was lying on the couch alone. They comforted me. I enjoyed wearing low-cut clothes and flaunting my breasts. [*Laughs.*] In fact, if I had only one piece of clothing to cover myself, it would be a pair of panties. I think most women would choose a bra, don't you?

Breasts are something men don't have, so they make a big fuss over them. I always felt inadequate when my husband read *Playboy*, because I was afraid he was comparing me unfavorably to the pictures. After I separated from him, I began to have a much better body image. I felt beautiful because my lover told me I was. I began to love my breasts more than ever right before my mastectomy. I'm only in my thirties and in three years I've gone through divorce, mastectomy, chemotherapy, menopause, and reconstruction.

The first cancer surgeon I consulted told me not to have reconstruction, but the one who operated on me mentioned it as an option. I couldn't bear to look at my mastectomy, and I didn't allow anyone else to see me nude either. My therapist suggested that I have sex with someone to feel more comfortable, but I felt deformed. My surgeon said that in the civilized world we don't mourn a lost part of the body, but in primitive cultures they hold funeral services for it. That makes a lot of sense to me.

I had read about reconstruction and seen pictures, so I did not expect perfection. However, I would have loved immediate reconstruction. The hospital I was in isn't doing that yet, and I only found out about it afterward. My plastic surgeon's office is run by a very understanding woman who's had two mastectomies and reconstruction.

Since my reconstruction, I've learned to care more for my body and to be most sensitive to physical frailty. My implant was too high, round, and firm in the beginning. At first I was afraid to go back to the surgeon, but he wanted to check it every so often. Last time he said, "This is not a good enough result. So we're doing it over with a 'local,' as an outpatient." I was glad that he recognized the problem. I thought I would just have to live with it that way. When I touch my breasts now, the skin over the implanted one feels cooler to me. I think that has to do with there not being as many nerves and blood vessels on top of it. It feels kind of nice, actually; my "air-conditioned" breast. [*Laughs.*] For a few months I could feel little pricks and jabs in the area. Then I got back some more sensation and, gradually, they've disappeared. Having a cleavage again means a great deal to me, and I'm always very much aware of having a breast again. Putting a bra on after reconstruction was the greatest.

ROSA

I had my mastectomy in 1977 at the hospital clinic. I knew about reconstruction a few years ago, because I saw it on television. I thought about doing it many times, but I wanted to see someone else who had done it first. When I asked the nurses, they told me they knew no one. Nobody explained anything, and when they did, the words were too big. My children, who are twenty-two and seventeen, gave me the courage to try it. I missed my breast very much. I was always busy covering up my chest if someone came to the door. When I told that to the doctor, he encouraged me, too. This year they did it with a flap from my back. I hate the scar on my back, though. Maybe if I knew about it before, I wouldn't bother myself about it, but I don't remember anybody telling me. My back sinks in where the flap was; not much, but a little. The doctor tells me that all the scars will lighten, so maybe the back one will, too. None of them show in my clothes, anyway.

Before the surgery, a friend told me that the implant could break and the insides would go to my heart. I decided then to ask the doctors instead of listening to friends. I would really like a nipple that sticks out more; this one is flat. You know the truth? [*Whispers.*] Deep inside myself, I am very happy that I did it, but I'm afraid that if I let the doctor see that, he will stop working on me to make it better.

ISABELLE

I'm in my early forties and I've worked as an administrator in the medical field for many years. I have three young children, and my husband is a long-term cancer survivor himself. I grew up in Europe in a very closed-off society, sexually speaking, so my pleasure in my breasts was only recognizable after my marriage.

I did self-examination and found the breast lump myself even though it was deep. It was 2¾ centimeters, but had been missed by the doctor in a recent checkup. I had so much denial going in for the biopsy that I practically skipped down the street to the hospital. When I awoke, my first gesture was with my right hand to my left breast. I had had a modified radical. My first words were "When can I have reconstruction?"

My husband has been extremely supportive, and I went into therapy right away. I've never mentioned the word "cancer" to the children, though. They coped beautifully, why should we talk about it? You know, out of my son's class of fifteen, five mothers have had breast cancer.

I had already seen many reconstructed women in my work. However, I had an elderly cancer surgeon who did not encourage reconstruction, saying that 90 percent of his patients did not have it done. After my mastectomy I found the sight of myself nude appalling. To me, reconstruction meant fighting back. My oncologist actually recommended the plastic surgeon. Also, my cousin is a plastic surgeon in San Francisco and had heard of the man recommended by my oncologist, as well as the RAM technique. For one year I spoke to everyone I knew who had reconstruction and went to interview about eight doctors. They either gave me very little time or threw out technical terms with no explanation. When I requested an explanation of one surgeon, he replied, "Oh, my nurse will write down the names for you." When I asked another doctor if it would be possible to undergo reconstruction while on chemotherapy, he asked, "Why on earth would you want to do that? You'll be putting on so much weight that your breast will be hanging down to your stomach!" My husband and I left the office in tears.

I then spent one very hot summer wearing my prosthesis. I

am a C cup, and the heat was absolute torture. I vowed that I would not go through a summer with a prosthesis again.

I had a generous stomach and chose the RAM procedure because it accomplishes a "tummy tuck" as well, so I'd get a new belly button out of it, too. [*Laughs.*] I also chose this method because I felt strongly about not having a foreign object in my body. However, I was one of the 10 percent who developed an abdominal infection, and I had to spend ten more days in the hospital on antibiotics. I did it the hard way, but I couldn't be happier.

Sexuality has been extended today; we now recognize many more years of sexual activity, and I felt that I would feel much more sexually whole with two breasts. And I do! The breast is superb! It is a little larger than my natural breast, but it will be "shaved down" when I go back to have the nipple-areola done. The surgery has created a protrusion on my abdomen, which I was not warned about, however, and my waistline has enlarged. I can no longer wear many of my old clothes. However, before my mastectomy, I had bought an exquisite lace dress which I couldn't wear without reconstruction. Now I can wear it again, and that gives me great satisfaction.

I feel that, after my experience, I have some good advice for other women. First, if you have no money for therapy, talk to your priest, your rabbi, etc.—anyone to give you an unemotional ear. Second, see plastic surgeons from different hospitals and of different opinions rather than just taking the opinion of one referring surgeon. That is because some hospitals will favor one technique and not another. You, however, should investigate all the options. I feel that I rushed into my mastectomy. If a woman takes two weeks to do research before her mastectomy, she is not risking anything, healthwise. She can do her reconstruction research then also, and it will give her a sense of control. She should also take a tape recorder with her to the consultations or an objective friend to make sure that she comprehends everything discussed. Sometimes the doctor will dictate a letter in front of the patient describing his recommendations to the referring physician. It may be possible to get a copy of that, if that is the case. Lastly, remember that elective surgery is so much harder because it is, finally, your decision.

DORIS

I'm single, in my early forties, and had always liked my bust line. Then, in 1978, I had a biopsy and mastectomy. I insisted on a two-stage procedure, even though there was a lot of opposition at that time. Most people thought I was crazy. I did a great deal of research on the subject before I went ahead with the mastectomy. Then, after the surgery, I started going to a postmastectomy group. I found that I was emotionally way ahead of the other women, though, because of all of my research. I felt that my doctor was the instrument who did it, but I was the control.

After the mastectomy I wouldn't even go out of my room without my prosthesis on. I live alone and I have very little family, but I became even more private than before. I began to do a great deal of research about reconstruction and I wrote a newspaper article which made use of my findings. My cancer surgeon was pessimistic at first, but when I saw him one year later, his attitude had changed because of the progress in the field. I had reconstruction using an implant in 1980. I think I might have had better results if I had waited even longer, but I'm very glad I did it. I didn't get my own bust line back, though. One of my friends had a beautiful figure but very unattractive breasts. Reconstruction was an improvement for her. For me it wasn't, and that hurts. But then I had a particularly nice bust line before. I could do it over, but I don't want to for money reasons, time out of work, etc. Many women I know even prefer bilateral mastectomy to reconstruction because they feel that at least then they have symmetry. Before my reconstruction my friend said, "I don't know about having a foreign object in your body." It made me wonder because I'm the kind of person who likes to take off my makeup as soon as I get home, you know? I like to be unencumbered, I like to take my bra off as soon as I can and I don't like tight belts, etc. So I kinda wondered if, after I got it in, would I want to pull it out? [*Laughs.*] But the great thing about it is, it helps you forget. You no longer identify with the cancer patient.

TONI

I'm thirty-nine, single, and the head of a typing pool in a big corporation. I found my own lump, and first I tried to treat myself with herb teas. I'm a big believer in that natural stuff. My cancer was the regular type, I guess. I only know of two types: the kind that's in one breast and the kind that spreads to the other breast. I was afraid to go to another doctor for a second opinion on the mastectomy. There was too much "red tape" to transfer the records, and I couldn't afford it anyway. I had a positive example in a very brave girl friend who had gone through it. I was actually more upset about the chemotherapy than about losing the breast. But once I accepted it, I didn't cry anymore.

For the first couple of years after the mastectomy, I was just happy that I recovered from the cancer. Then I got more unhappy about losing the breast, in terms of my future relationships. I hadn't been involved with how I looked during chemotherapy, but afterward I became upset about my body. I never had any reason to be inhibited before and now I did. But it still didn't stop me from having relationships. If I'm still attractive otherwise, then what's the big deal? Why wouldn't they accept me because I just have one breast? I really just wanted a breast to wear low-cut clothes again, but it didn't mean much in terms of relationships. I have a problem, anyway, getting into heavy relationships with men; mentally and emotionally that is, but not physically. Even without the breast, I wasn't afraid to go with anyone. I'm not shy that way.

I go mostly with blue-collar workers and they're not sensitive that way. If you're gonna go with an artist, they might have more trouble with it; they're delicate, squeamish. A fireman deals with life and death all the time, he sees everything. He's not gonna think that one breast is a big deal. I don't think the problem is only the way a woman feels about herself. It also depends on the men you deal with. I always go for macho types. It doesn't bother them, they don't bat an eye. Other women have told me that the men are the problem, too. They just couldn't take it. I had only one bad experience, with a musician whose sister had died of breast cancer. When I told him about mine, he became very upset, but I thought that it was more about the cancer than the breast.

I first heard about reconstruction when my brother-in-law suggested it during a visit to the hospital. He had seen it on a TV program. I took a while to make up my mind, and then my HIP program found me a surgeon. He's a very creative person who gave me choices and was not hard and fast in his rules. I needed a flap procedure because my skin was so tight. The mastectomy scar was very high because they took a lot of skin. I was told that, with the latissimus dorsi flap, the implant might shift, so I chose the gluteus. I wanted reconstruction to be whole-feeling again, and for vanity, not practical, purposes. I didn't use the RAM because I might want to have children. Also, making a new navel didn't thrill me. The gluteus flap sounded frightening at first. I was very nervous that the arteries and veins wouldn't be connected right, but then I thought, "He's so famous, I'm very lucky to have him." I wanted to read about reconstruction, but I couldn't find any books.

I couldn't enjoy my new breast at first because I had several complications. I was hospitalized for longer than usual, but it wasn't the surgeon's fault. Those complications are very rare and could happen to anyone. It was the way my body reacted.

I always felt inadequate and self-conscious in high school because of my small breasts. I didn't feel like I was a woman. The other girls became women, but I stayed a girl because I was so flat. Now I'm happy that he made my breast small. If I had an implant, I guess I'd have fewer scars, but they'll fade. It's not exactly like the other breast, it's a little bigger. In a few months he's going to halve the other nipple and use the upper inner thigh for the areola. He also wants to "tuck" the other breast a little then. The back donor site is sunken in, and that disappoints me. I'm afraid it might be noticeable in tight pants or a bathing suit, but I'm still happy I did it. The only really bad thing is that I was pressured into going back to work sooner than I felt I could. My family, though, has been very supportive.

I had realistic expectations and I can't understand women who are against reconstruction because they won't get their own breast back. I would tell them to be realistic and then, if they really want it, do it. I found support groups to be really helpful. Everyone looked so good, so healthy, and it helped to talk. I had felt like a real loser, losing my breast. They had lost them, too, but they didn't look like losers, so I figured maybe I didn't either.

JESSICA

Okay, let's see . . . I design clothes, I'm in my mid-thirties, and I'm divorced with three children. My mother had cancer of the breast, too. I discovered my own breast lump at the end of a love affair, but my lover couldn't be supportive when he heard it was cancer. I had the mastectomy in the spring of '82 and another male friend came to be with me. I made the decision to do the mastectomy for life reasons. Anything else was a gamble. My surgeon said to me, "You will have a mastectomy, but you will be reconstructed." That was the first time I ever heard of reconstruction. He gave me an example of a famous woman who had successful reconstruction and I held on to that for dear life. When I asked my breast surgeon if it would look perfect, he said, "With dim lights and a little camouflage, yes." I guess camouflage meant a see-through nightie. But when my ex-husband was called by the doctor to tell him about my lump, his answer was "Tell her this won't make me come back."

I was able to look at my chest right away after mastectomy and I felt comfortable clothed with a prosthesis. In fact, I went right back to work. My life had changed, but it wasn't as devastating as I'd expected. About one month after the surgery I thought, "I'm so tired. Do I really need reconstruction? I don't think I want my body 'mushied' around with anymore." I had gotten used to the breast loss a bit. But I went ahead and researched reconstruction very thoroughly. I wanted to go ahead with it so that I could wear revealing clothes and to avoid complex explanations in intimate situations. I also felt that if I didn't do it quickly, I wouldn't do it at all and would always wonder if I should have. Some plastic surgeons' photographs scared me, while others gave me false hope. My father had discouraged me from having the reconstruction, saying, "Why ask for more problems?" He told me about all the mastectomized women he had known and been attracted to. A surgeon friend even told me that he finds a mastectomy rather appealing but not a reconstruction.

When the time came, I decided to use a plastic surgeon who did nothing but breast surgery. I figured that he would have the most experience possible in terms of problems, successes, etc. We used an implant filled with saline solution. The thing that made me most nervous was being awake in the operating room. The doctor was very understanding; he told me that if I was too nervous to go ahead, I could go home if I wanted to. He said that one of his patients had gone home three times before she went through with it. After the surgery I had a problem with some bleeding around one implant, and a short repair procedure was necessary. That was done as an outpatient under a local anesthetic. I only felt pressure, no pain. I am terrified of general anesthesia, so it was fine with me. The surgeon talked to me and made me laugh all during the procedure. That made me feel much better. There was an anesthesiologist standing by if I wanted it, but I would encourage any woman to have a "local" if possible. I think that a sense of humor and not being afraid to laugh is what gets you through all this, you know. A lot of people think you're not supposed to laugh because it's about cancer, but I think if you didn't laugh, you'd just cry all the time.

Even though I had some problems with my reconstruction, I am thrilled with my new breast! It "works" perfectly and I think it's beautiful. I think I might even like it better than the old one. I immediately bought a plunging-neckline blouse and spend my time bending over a lot. [*Laughs.*] I think that it relieves other people to see my reconstructed breast and to see me looking so good. It hasn't erased the cancer experience, though.

Reconstruction relieved the feeling of tightness in my chest. I was told, however, not to exert myself for one month; no opening windows, not even pulling down a shade. If I ever needed a second mastectomy, I would console myself with the option of reconstructing a perfect "match." I realized that my expectations were unrealistic the first time. I expected an exact duplicate of my natural breast. I also feel that reconstruction is encouraging for my daughters to see so they know what can be done for women who have had mastectomies.

I'm still deciding about the second stage, the nipple-areola graft, but that's just a two-to-three-hour visit to the hospital, a very short procedure, and a local anesthetic. My surgeon does not "tuck" the other breast unless absolutely necessary; he's into keeping what you've got nice.

One man that I dated while I was breastless was very attentive then, but he's a little "spooked" by the implant. Another man thinks it's fabulous, but then, he's sexually very confident. He calls it "the breast of a sex goddess." On a date, talking about life experiences and especially about profound ones, it's very difficult not to share this one. It's always in the front of my mind, especially since it's changed my attitudes about so many things. It's hard not to talk about it. I worry about when to say something. I think it always has to be dealt with in advance of intimacy whether you've had a reconstruction or just the mastectomy, even though I think that your sexuality starts way before your clothes are taken off. My worst fantasy before reconstruction was that a man would touch the mastectomy side by accident and faint or run away or something. I wouldn't have been comfortable then having any man touch me on my flat side; I always kept a T-shirt on in bed.

I have a really sweet new man now, and when we started to get involved, I said, "You know, I was very sick a couple of years ago, but I'm fine now." He said, "The important thing is that you're well now." I took hold of his hand and asked if he would like to touch my new breast. He did and said, "That feels wonderful! I didn't know anything like that was possible." I had this sudden fear then that when he touched the real one it wouldn't feel as good. [*Laughs.*] The reconstruction made all the difference in the world at that moment, even though I knew, intellectually, that he was interested in me whether I had one breast or six.

My advice to other women who want breast reconstruction would be to have it done as soon as possible. If you wait too long, you might not do it, and it's wonderful to have. Also, if you can't have a private nurse, ask a friend to come stay with you for support and TLC. The nurses are very overworked and too busy with critically ill people to be very attentive. With the implants, it's only a two-day stay at the most, but that first day does hurt. Most important, find someone who's a good example, a woman who has done it and can "talk you through" the experience. Look, I'm very happy I had it done, but then I'm on this side of it; I'm finished.

EUNICE

I didn't even tell my six children about my mastectomy because I felt self-conscious. I didn't tell anybody. My mother is old and I don't have any other relatives. I just took all my troubles to God. I only confided in Him. I found the lump myself and did the mastectomy because life comes first. I had to have chemotherapy, too. I missed my breast very much. I just didn't feel like my old self.

I had never heard of reconstruction. The doctors said nothing, but I was waiting in the clinic to go in for my mastectomy and the lady next to me asked what I was there for. She told me she had both her breasts off. She wrote something on a piece of paper and handed it to me, saying, "Now you make sure you show this to the doctor when you go in." The word was "Reconstruct." I did like she said even though I wasn't sure what it meant.

After my mastectomy my daughter said to me, "Momma, whatever is wrong with you, you're takin' it good, and you don't bother nobody with it." That made me very proud. [*Smiles.*] I didn't worry about hugging my children after the mastectomy, because that's not my style. I just tell them all the time that I love them. We don't go in much for hugging.

I never married, but the same man is the father of all my children. I didn't think to tell him about all this because he has a "split personality": one when he's sober and another one when he's drinking. I was afraid that, when he'd be drunk, he'd use it against me and my kids. When I'm all back to myself and strong again, maybe I'll share it with him. I have an implant now and I'm very happy. I feel like my old self again. I can forget now that I was sick.

VICTORIA

I'm married with one teenager and I had a radical mastectomy in 1977. Fortunately, I didn't require any chemotherapy or radiation. I wasn't able to be very open with my son, however. The time to talk about it just never seemed right. I was always considered a very attractive actress, and I was terrified of losing my sexuality. I even thought, for a while after the mastectomy, that people at work were ridiculing me behind my back. I thought that, because I had lost my breast, I had also lost all sexual power and drive. My breasts were very critical in terms of lovemaking and achieving orgasm, and because I refused to acknowledge my chest at all after the mastectomy, I became frigid. After all, I still had one breast in perfect "working order," but if I thought about that one it only reminded me that the other one was gone. I never could keep hold of the fact that the cancer was a real threat to my life. Instead, I focused totally on the loss of the breast. I didn't allow my husband to see me naked after the mastectomy, even though he was very supportive. I had seen a woman at the health club walking around naked with a radical mastectomy and I found it shocking and ugly. I even made love with my bra on, though my husband was not at all reluctant to touch the breastless side. I wouldn't even touch myself; my stomach would "clutch" at the sight of my chest. It was very neat surgery, just a flat chest with one pink scar line. It just wasn't "me."

I knew I wanted reconstruction from the beginning. I had read a book about it in which the writer set a good example. My husband's attitude about reconstruction was that I should do whatever would make me happy; if I was happy, he said that he would be. I talked to two doctors, plastic surgeons. One recommended implants, but I was nervous about infection and shifting. I had also heard wonderful things about the gluteal flap operation. Even though I desperately wanted to repair the mastectomy, I took a long time to decide. I read as much as I could find on reconstruction and interviewed women who had done it. The surgeon told me that the reconstructed breast would be fuller and higher than the other one, but it was even more so. He said that he could halve the other nipple, but I was terrified of losing sensation. The first nipple graft caved in a little, so he decided to take the grafts again from my earlobe. At the same time, he reshaped the reconstructed side and "tucked" the natural breast for symmetry. I lost no feeling at all on that side, so that was great! I remember I was so happy with the results when I woke up. The flap site is not even noticeable in a bathing suit. The *best* part is that when the normal breast is stimulated now, I feel some erotic stimulation on the reconstructed side, too. That may be psychological, I don't know, but I don't care what the explanation is, I'm just going to enjoy it. [*Laughs.*] I feel that I'm really finished now with the whole experience. The strange thing is that before I had cancer I always assumed that everyone but me had beautiful breasts that were equal in size. But the other day a friend told me about a new bra named "Nobody's Perfect" which capitalizes on the fact that most women's breasts are asymmetrical to begin with, something that many women use as a complaint about their surgery. I realized that part of my problem was that I had a fantasy of being given perfect, symmetrical breasts as a reward for having had cancer.

I think women should discuss implants as well as the other options very thoroughly and then make the decision best for them. As for immediate reconstruction, I'm against it, because I feel that you need time first to recover from the whole idea of the disease.

ELLEN

I'm forty-three and a widow and I'm a senior vice-president of a large corporation. After a biopsy in 1982 I did a lot of research for about a month before I decided on a mastectomy instead of a lumpectomy with radiation. I visited several prominent specialists on both sides of the controversy, and after studying all of the options, I made my choice. I did not really trust lumpectomy-radiation to handle the disease as effectively as mastectomy, and I worried about the possibility of poor cosmetic results and the long-term risks of radiation. I was much more comfortable with the concept of mastectomy and reconstruction.

My cancer surgeon advised leaving the nipple, but I wanted a second opinion. The next surgeon felt strongly that, with an intraductal carcinoma, the nipple should not be left because of the risk of cancer cells in that area as well. I consulted a plastic surgeon before the mastectomy and he preferred not leaving the nipple, because he feels he can achieve a more satisfactory symmetry without it. I first heard about reconstruction from an old friend whom I had watched go through mastectomy and reconstruction. Her experience helped me tremendously by setting an example for me to follow. She helped me through my odyssey, and now I'm doing the same for another friend. The passing on of experience is a vital issue here.

My cancer surgeon recommended the plastic surgeon. I chose him because he did only breast surgery and I liked the hospital. It was the same one where the biopsy and mastectomy were done and I felt comfortable there. He also said, "I can do a good job for you."

My parents are quite old and my mother is ill, so I wanted to spare them my disease and reconstruction. I told them that I was going on a business trip, which I do frequently, anyway. I was also afraid that they would make me feel too sorry for myself, and talking about it with family and friends would have meant facing my feelings. I had a therapist for that and I didn't have to worry about her feelings. I felt I could handle the loss in terms of keeping a secret. Besides, I was concerned about my job. I had not been with the firm very long, and I was afraid it might change the way the management thought of me. Perhaps not, but I was afraid to take the chance. It was important to me that no one, with the exception of that one friend, know what I was going through. I've always been private to a fault, and this was no exception.

The mastectomy site was actually much less grotesque than I had imagined. It was very tidy and I was surprised at how ungruesome it was. But it was still a constant reminder of the disease. I had no sexual involvements after the mastectomy and before the reconstruction; no "auditioning." I felt, at that time, that the men in my life were not appropriate choices for such a sensitive issue.

I expected complications with reconstruction, but I also expected a good job. I had no complications at all and the breast is absolutely wonderful! It's soft, pliable, and a very good match with the other one. One thing happened in the hospital that I wish I had known about before. In the middle of the night, after surgery, I woke up and touched my new breast to make sure I hadn't dreamed the whole thing. I was horrified to feel a lump. Too groggy to call the nurse, I suffered through the rest of the night only to learn that it was just a postoperative drain. I had thought, "Just my luck! I come in for reconstruction and I'm punished with another cancer!"

Reconstruction isn't such an interruption of your life either. I checked in to the hospital one afternoon, was operated on the next morning, and went home the following morning. I was a little washed out for a few days, but I went back to work within the week. The anesthesia is what really knocks you out most. The oblique mastectomy scar will fade, and the only small disappointment is that the scar under the breast is healing with keloids, so it's bumpy. If I'm exposed, I'm self-conscious about the scar but not the breast. The new breast matches the other one exactly in a bra (you can't see the scar then, of course) and I can sleep on it with no difficulty. It's easier to sleep on the small implants anyway. Larger than a B cup, it's less comfortable, they tell me. Anyway, I'm going ahead with the final phase for the most natural appearance.

The option of reconstruction from the beginning made the cancer much easier to endure, and after plastic surgery I felt much further away from the disease. The breast replacement was to satisfy an aesthetic need and to negate the everyday physical reminder. I like it for *myself,* for nobody else! Also, I always felt positive about my small breasts and now I have them both back.

My advice to other women would be to shop around and to use an experienced plastic surgeon who does breasts exclusively, if possible. Remember, pass on your experience to the next person. It does so much to alleviate so many anxieties.

LISA

I'm single and thirty-two and have a really good job in advertising. I was a tomboy when I was an adolescent and I honestly didn't want to grow breasts. They got in my way in sports. Later, I was still not that focused on my breasts. They were just there, that's all. They weren't that critical to my sexual stimulation.

My mother had died of cancer, and when I learned that I had breast cancer my attitude was "Take it out, kill it!" I felt like I had maggots inside me or something.

In the recovery room after the mastectomy, my surgeon suggested reconstruction. He told me that he had operated on me with that in mind, but he advised me to wait one year. The thought of reconstruction kept me going, but I still missed that part of me terribly. I had never had to give clothing much thought before. You know, if I saw something I liked, I bought it. After the mastectomy I couldn't wear a lot of my nicest clothes, even with a prosthesis. I couldn't wear scoop necklines because, when I bent over, the flatness over the top of the bra showed. I felt like Miss Prim in my high-necked dresses. Also, I was quite large-breasted, and with the weight on one side and not the other, unless I wore my prosthesis all day long, I could feel the strain in my back. I avoided dating all during my "breastless period": too many explanations. I was too worried about their reactions.

I had never met anyone with a mastectomy until I started my year of researching reconstruction. I joined a support group and interviewed three or four plastic surgeons. The women in that group gave me good perspective. None of them thought that their reconstructions were totally perfect, but the others considered them wonderful. I've found that to be true all over. It's like knowing that your living room needs painting, but it looks perfect to your guests. They go home and say, "Boy, their place was beautiful! We better do something about ours."

I was really well informed about the procedure of reconstruction and found it less complicated than I'd expected. My other breast was at great risk also, and I was advised to do a prophylactic mastectomy. I would have needed reduction surgery on it to have made a match, so I decided to have it removed about one year after the first mastectomy. A bilateral reconstruction sounded good to me because I wouldn't have to be worried about asymmetry, and I liked the idea of never having to wear a bra again. My family was very supportive, but my sister felt that I should leave well enough alone. She had read an article that emphasized the problems with reconstruction, most of which occur very rarely, but didn't give equal time to the positives. As for me, I couldn't wait to get back to the way I felt before all of this cancer business, to the clothing I liked, and the freedom from bulky prostheses.

My internist gave me the names of several plastic surgeons, but I liked the first one on the list. I had tight, thin skin, so he inserted temporary expanders, which were not that natural-looking. But, emotionally, it was still a thrill to have them there. They weren't part of me and the expanding process was a bit uncomfortable, but I knew it was just temporary. I could feel the valve just under the skin for the expander and, luckily, the doctor told me it was there or I would have thought I'd grown another lump. When the skin stretched after a few weeks, double-lumen implants were inserted. The first day I was really pretty uncomfortable, but I took pain medication and by the next day I was tired but fine. Actually, I didn't find reconstruction as painful as mastectomy. It seems to be different for everybody. I'm now a B cup, smaller than I was before, and very happy. I love pretty lingerie even though I don't need a bra anymore. When I do wear one, the ones with the stretch cups are the best because they mold to the individual breast. I've really lost the feeling of doom and gloom that I associated with having cancer. I started dating again and I met someone who's very sensitive to my situation. Reconstruction made all the difference in the world! I even decided not to do the second stage now because I don't want to give up my daily tennis game with my "honey." I guess I value the contour over the nipple.

I doubt that I would have appreciated a breast that was immediately reconstructed. I think I would still have expected my own breast back and been disappointed. On the other hand, that time in between was pretty painful, so maybe. . . . My advice would be to ask the surgeon every question you can think of and take notes! You'll have more control over the decisions. Be prepared for variable results, but definitely do it.

GRACE

I'm seventy and five times a grandma. In 1979 I had a bilateral mastectomy. Afterward I missed my breasts something terrible. Then, last year, I went to visit my friend Gloria's daughter, who had her breast reconstructed. I drove three hundred miles alone just to get a look at it! [*Laughs.*] Well, that did it! I went to ask my cancer surgeon if I had "missed the boat" because of my age. He said that had nothing to do with it and he really encouraged me to have reconstruction, too. He gave me different choices, but I wanted the simplest all around, so we picked the implants. The choices made me feel like I was in charge for a change, though. My husband was against the reconstruction, felt I didn't need it. The more he said, "You don't have to do this for me" and "I don't know why you're bothering," the madder I got! Finally I said, "For heaven's sake, I am not doing it for *you*, I'm doing it for *me!*" [*Laughs.*] He never said anything against it again.

Whenever I've had anesthesia, I'm just thrilled to be alive when I wake up. I guess that's one reason why immediate reconstruction is great; you don't have to "go under" twice.

My cancer surgeon worked as a team with the plastic surgeon. They talked about me before the reconstruction. They also worked with a woman psychiatrist. I was very well prepared, especially the emotional part. They told me exactly what to expect every step of the way.

I'm really happy with these implants. In fact, I appreciate them a lot more than I ever did the old ones. [*Laughs.*] One is a little firmer, so I call it my "masculine" breast. Right now I don't feel I need nipples. I met a woman the other day who had a double mastectomy and didn't want a reconstruction. That amazed me! But she seemed perfectly fine about it.

My Major Medical paid almost all of my doctor's fee after I wrote them a letter saying how much this surgery meant to me. Now that I had it all rebuilt, I'm a changed person. I even walk different now. At one point I was advised to find a support group. But then I said to myself, "Woman, you don't have cancer, you *had it!* You're your old feisty self again!"

ANNE

When I had my radical mastectomy, I was sixty-five. I was just eager to get the disease out of my body and I didn't trust anything less to do it thoroughly. Also, my type of cancer, though tiny, was not the right sort for lumpectomy. I couldn't have lived with wondering if we had done enough anyway.

At that point, I had been married for forty-five years and my husband said that reconstruction was not important to him. We would joke about the fact that I had such tiny breasts before that a tiny bit less would hardly matter. I knew he loved me for many reasons, the least of which was my breast.

I've heard a great deal about reconstruction, but it's not for me. My daughter had a bilateral mastectomy and reconstruction, and for her I think it's important to rebuild her breasts. Her job puts her in the public eye and also, at forty, she's still young. Besides, when I had my surgery, no one I knew had had reconstruction or even heard of it, so it never occurred to me to consider it. I felt I was too old then and now I feel I'm certainly too old [seventy]. The cancer was such a horrible experience for me that I never want to see the inside of a hospital again. It's not the physical discomfort that bothers me about surgery; that's short-lived, according to my daughter, and the pain medication is very effective. I just think, "Why should I do that? I'm old. I don't think about my breasts anymore. At my age I don't have to be interested in those things." I hate my body now, though. I find my scar ugly and avoid looking at it. I never touch it either. It feels awful; sends shivers up my spine. The radical left a big depression on my chest and under my arm, so my clothing choice is limited. I guess if immediate reconstruction had been available to me then, I wouldn't be so angry about my body now. It's a pity, really. Everyone used to say that I had a lovely figure. They were right, too.

JO

I have a very active life: a busy career in architecture, a husband, and four kids (actually, four grown-ups now). I had my second breast removed, prophylactically, six years ago, many years after a radical mastectomy of the first at age twenty-nine. I would be lying if I didn't say, "Hey, wouldn't it be nice to be sitting here with two breasts?" but I couldn't put myself through that. With a radical on one side, I'd need a flap, and on the other side, an implant. It would be a question of many hours on that table. In the beginning I felt worse about it, but I've gotten so used to my body this way.

I am, and always have been, very open with my husband and children about my body. At home, my prostheses are often draped over a chair when I don't want the bother of putting on a bra. If the kids are having friends over, I'll ask them how they feel about my not wearing the prostheses. They'll always say something like, "Don't worry about us, Mom. It's not important." After many years I guess you could say we've all made a comfortable adjustment to my being breastless.

8

Professional Counseling: Ear Lending, Ear Bending

So many times during my interviews with women, they stressed the need for emotional support in making treatment decisions and in wrestling with the psychological turmoil following breast surgery. The word "isolation" came up most frequently in describing the feelings of a mastectomized woman, and "I wish I knew someone who's done it" was expressed by those hesitant about taking the step toward reconstruction. Whether counseling took a private or group form, very rarely did a woman complain that it was a negative experience. I visited and interviewed several types of professionals dedicated to helping cancer patients toward recovery.

For regional counseling by a social worker, singly or in groups, you can consult the National Association of Social Workers's *Directory of Professional Social Workers*, obtained through any local hospital. That will ensure you a professional counselor and provide you with the names and addresses of those located in your area. The registry would specify therapists who have specialized experience, and in the majority of states there is reimbursement for counseling from most insurance companies. It's a good idea to jot down several names and talk with a few before making your final decision. As in any relationship, chemistry is an important factor, and it's wise to choose someone you feel you can like and trust. I'll try to give you an idea of how group counseling works and how counselors can help you.

Patricia (Pat) Sawyer, A.C.S.W. (Academy of Certified Social Workers), works at the Institute of Rehabilitation Medicine at New York University Medical Center. Soft-spoken, with a pixie haircut and a generous smile, Pat has undergone bilateral mastectomy but not reconstruction. She offers eight weekly sessions for postmastectomy patients at the medical center and explained that her group covers all problems associated with breast cancer. There is no charge and the group is funded by a grant from Dr. Howard Rusk in memory of his late wife. The focus is on the concerns of the individual members. On occasion, guest speakers are invited to talk on related subjects, including reconstruction.

I spoke to Pat at length about her work with these women. One of her main concerns is that there aren't enough places for a woman to be able to talk, to open up. She feels, however, that groups are not for everyone; sometimes individual counseling makes a woman more comfortable. She emphasized that social workers have more experience with medically related issues than most other therapists. They often get to see and meet the patient's family in the hospital or at home. That way, they can consider the patient in her surroundings and treat the entire issue as to how it relates to the patient's world; e.g., is she feeling pressure from family, friends, or work? Postmastectomy women often report that, since their surgery, they don't even go to the same supermarket or beauty parlor. Women need help with the psychological issue most, when all of the physical caring related to the mastectomy is through. It's difficult, Pat explained, for a great many surgeons to deal with the emotionality of the issue. They have to maintain their objectivity; the need for them to view the body as a machine is jeopardized by their emotional involvement. That is why she believes in a "middleman" to deal with the emotional part of recovery. However, she has found that it is extremely difficult to get groups like hers started. The "old guard" component of the medical community is not used to this way of thinking. They feel that it is sometimes dangerous to open up feelings, and tend to think of the patient in terms of physical recuperation only. Rare inpatient groups at hospitals are more successful, since they are made up of a captive audience. Because there aren't funds for support groups like hers, a lot of social workers have become just "travel agents": someone who decides, with the surgeon, when a patient is ready to leave the hospital.

Pat's advice to women looking for a plastic surgeon is first get a recommendation from your cancer surgeon and then get a totally different view. If possible, consult someone at another hospital than the one in which you had the cancer surgery. With the surgeon's recommendation, it is more likely to be his colleague at the same medical center, who will often hold similar views. If you consult someone at another center, at least there will be a range of opinion even though you may find that your final choice of doctor is the same as your surgeon's.

Pat feels that many lives are saved because of the option of reconstruction, but she disagrees with proponents of immediate reconstruction. She feels that the patient needs time to make an adjustment to what has happened to her body and her psyche as a result of cancer.

With the group's permission, I sat in on one of the weekly sessions. Pat feels strongly that it is critical that a support group have professional personnel to lead it. Best of all, there should be access to a medical center or physicians. The greatest danger, she feels, is that every layperson considers herself an expert if she's had the cancer experience. This can mean that she imposes her misinformation as well as information on the group, which can be dangerous. It is a difficult enough period for women even with the correct data. Women are often fearful that, if they let out their feelings, they will not regain control; but if they don't let them out, it is even more difficult to make appropriate decisions either on the initial surgery or on reconstruction. The term "breakdown" is generally thought of as a negative and a weakness when really, Pat points out, it is just reacting normally to stress.

She feels it's best if the women's partners can join in to provide information as well. She has opened up the group to the partners, but finds that the message often doesn't get home, because a woman is sometimes fearful of hearing her partner's concerns. The partner has an adjustment to make, too, but the patient often feels that it's only her problem. At times the partner may avoid touching or talking about the mastectomy side because he thinks that will be more protective toward the woman, and she, in turn, assumes that he doesn't care or is repulsed by it. What results is a communications barrier.

Pat believes that adult children would benefit from the counseling as well. Women often make the mistake of assuming the feelings of their family members without ever discussing the situation openly. Sharing it makes an even more special family relationship. It sets an example for the children to follow in their own lives.

Gay couples she has counseled have much the same problems adjusting to breastlessness as heterosexuals. Pat believes in being frank with all of her women and tells them, "After cancer, nothing in your life is going to be the same. When you go on, it's to something new. It can be better, but it can't ever be the same."

The meeting I attended was held in the "doll room" at the Rusk Institute of New York University Medical Center. Six women attended, all of whom were currently receiving or had just completed a course of chemotherapy. The youngest woman present, whom I judged to be in her early thirties, had undergone simultaneous mastectomy and reconstruction and had just finished chemotherapy. None of the other women had been reconstructed. We sat around a polished wood table in the comfortably furnished room, hundreds of gaily costumed dolls looking down at us from floor-to-ceiling shelves. Pat told me they were gifts from all over the world to Dr. Rusk in recognition of his work in rehabilitation.

Some of the women remained silent throughout the discussion on breast reconstruction, but the rest ranged from mildly curious to very interested. One woman said, "It's nice to know there's a choice. It's a gift to find that I could rebuild a radical mastectomy even if I never did it." On the subject of immediate reconstruction another said, "That kind of appeals to me. It's easier to be a coward once in terms of undergoing general anesthesia." As we ended the discussion, I stood up to leave and one woman who had remained quiet throughout the meeting asked shyly, "Would you show us yours?" Unaccustomed to group exposure, I said I'd be glad to display my reconstructed breasts to any interested women, one at a time, in the ladies' room. She was delighted. That's what I mean by positive example.

Pat introduced me to Dr. Stephen L. Gumport, a white-haired cancer surgeon at New York University Medical Center and medical director of the Gladys Houx Rusk Cancer Rehabilitation Service, who impressed me with his gentle manner and soft-spoken analysis of his patients' postmastectomy reactions. He estimated that, up until now, only one out of twenty or thirty women chose to undergo reconstruction, but he acknowledged that, most often, the women to whom he spoke were immediately postmastectomy and felt they couldn't face another procedure. Also, they knew very little about the subject. With time and knowledge, he agreed that attitude would very likely change.

Dr. Jerome Urban had told me earlier that many of his patients who could not face mastectomy without the option of reconstruction later decide not to go through the plastic surgery, saying that they are interested only in remaining disease-free. He told me that he always mentions reconstruction to his patients, believing that it's a good option, definitely very nice to have, but not necessarily for everyone. Many women are not as interested in reconstruction opportunities while they are still concerned with the eradication of the disease. Once they become reasonably confident that it has been eradicated, they begin to focus more on their altered bodies.

Dr. Gumport said, "It's incredible to me that women actually believe that we, as surgeons, are anxious to remove a breast. There is a great deal of other surgery that I could do. My heart's desire would be to tell a woman that I didn't have to remove her breast. . . . Nothing would make most surgeons happier than to have a method develop that would not require mastectomy, but we're not there yet." He commented, looking at Pat and me, that both of us had done extremely well with what we each decided to do, one to reconstruct and one not to. He smiled and said, "You certainly can't tell who chose what by your faces. You're both examples of excellent rehabilitation."

Virginia McCarthy is a psychiatric social worker who, in addition to a private practice, leads postmastectomy groups under the auspices of the Ninety-second Street YWHA in New York City. She has not had a personal experience with breast cancer, but provided some interesting insights into the attitudes of the group's women toward reconstruction. She sees these women for a ten-week period of counseling, not limited to immediately postmastectomy. She estimated that roughly 55 percent of her group members are negative about reconstruction, with the remaining 45 percent in favor of it. Most of the women express an ambivalence about wearing the external prosthesis, but, even so, the majority are very fearful of being hospitalized for surgery again. Virginia observed that this attitude is more prevalent immediately postmastectomy and changes, she thinks, with time. Some staunch feminists are against reconstruction, claiming that "a real woman doesn't need it." She has noticed that mentioning reconstruction to the group can be anxiety-provoking, but not mentioning it can also be disturbing. It elicits violent reactions for and against the topic. Some of the women recently operated on can't deal with it; they're in too much psychic pain. Their basic concern is life. She also questions how many decisions are made on the basis of what a woman thinks she is expected to do or feel. "Some women truly don't know what they feel. If you have denied the importance of the loss, then, when reconstruction is mentioned, you have to question yourself and face your feelings. You would have to acknowledge the pain; i.e., 'Yes, I feel the loss. Yes, I want the breast back.' Many women have not been able to come to terms with their feelings of pain and loss in this area." In her group, Virginia feels that what the women have to say to one another is of prime importance in the recovery process.

I spent a memorable afternoon at New York Hospital with Amy Chou, a clinical nursing specialist who, for the past twelve years, has been working exclusively with women facing breast surgery. She is petite, with long, straight dark hair and large dark eyes framed by huge eyeglasses. At first glance she appears to be no older than a teenager, but, as we sat in the empty nursing office at twilight, her maturity and experience were revealed in her passionate interest in her work.

I asked Amy how she came to work in this capacity. She replied that she has always been clinically oriented and after obtaining her master's degree she returned to work for a very dynamic department head who said, "Amy, do whatever you can to improve patient care." She became involved in giving patients care and support before surgery. Within the first week she met two women, one facing a definite mastectomy and the other a strong candidate for the same. The strong reactions of both these women to the news of breast cancer made such an impact on her that she made the decision to involve herself totally in this area.

When women are admitted to the hospital with breast lumps, Amy talks and walks them through the surgical experience as well as telephoning many of them at home afterward. She becomes very attached to "her women" and they to her. She also follows them through reconstruction whenever possible, and feels privileged to have a department head who encourages her and with whom she works closely. In a hospital newsletter, Amy is quoted as saying: "I began to realize how difficult the operation was. Physically, it's relatively simple and complications are rare. But the patients' emotional needs are immense. There is so little time. Usually just one day between admission and surgery, and the average stay is about seven days. Within that time, a woman must face the initial surgery, the immediate loss of a breast and the diagnosis of a malignancy, the verdict as to whether she will need additional treatment, and the question of whether she will be able to have reconstructive surgery."

Amy introduces the subject of reconstruction when she first talks to a new patient about possible mastectomy. She admitted, "I know that I do have the advantage of being in a big city like New York and in a hospital like this. Actually, very often I have to say to myself, 'Amy, you are really in a very unique situation.' Most of our patients here are already aware of reconstruction, and most of our doctors have already discussed it with them. So, unless a woman has very advanced disease, she can consider reconstruction as a very viable option to discuss even before her mastectomy."

Recently she had a patient near eighty who refused to sign for permission to remove the breast. Finally, after being reassured, over and over, that she could return for a reconstruction, she agreed. Amy has a current patient in her seventies who is eagerly looking forward to reconstruction. Amy says, "Especially in the current controversy over lumpectomy and mastectomy, if a woman is advised to definitely consider mastectomy for adequate disease control, then the option of reconstruction is very important. Women sometimes make the mistake of thinking that if I am a surgical nurse and their doctor is a surgeon, then all we want to do is cut. But all we really want to do is save a life. At times I find that a patient responds more readily to me than to their doctor because I, too, am a woman. I come into the picture and I don't talk about the frightening statistics. I just point out that their health is the most important consideration. Reconstruction has become so successful now. As recently as two years ago I was still leery about it, but not now."

Amy told me that she is now seeing younger women coming in with breast cancers. She believes this is partly because women are more aware of being examined regularly and doctors are now more aware of the necessity of being watchful earlier. With some of her patients, the only thing getting them through the cancer surgery is the thought of reconstruction. For those women, she talks about it at great length, pre-op, post-op, all the way through. For those who don't feel that it is an important issue, she doesn't force it. However, Amy doesn't find that being close to the cancer experience keeps a woman from necessarily wanting to talk about planning her reconstruction. Some women are opposed from the start on the grounds that the breast is really not that important to them and that their husbands don't care. Others say, "Let me get through this first and see what the pathology report says about further treatment. Let me take one step at a time." One patient of Amy's swore that she had no interest in rehabilitative surgery at all and was in psychotherapy for another problem. The therapist encouraged her to have reconstruction, and she was amazed at how thrilled she was that she had done it. For patients who resist the idea, she usually says, "Well, you can't have it for a while anyway, so that gives you a period of time to think about it and to determine how you really feel. You don't have to say no, you don't have to say yes. Just know that it is available to you if you want it." She says that it is most important for women to know that they have an option.

One patient Amy will never forget chose to do a lumpectomy but, to the day she went home, was still questioning her decision. Amy says, "She kept repeating, 'I want someone to tell me what to do.' But no one can make that decision for her. They can only advise her."

Amy asks her patients to notify her when they are coming back for reconstruction, and then she follows them through that procedure as well. To her knowledge, not one other hospital has a nurse in a job like hers, and it is so badly needed. In cases where supporters like herself are not readily available, she recommends that a woman interested in reconstruction inquire about it through a nurse in her hospital or a social service individual in her area. She could also specify a Reach to Recovery volunteer once she is home from the hospital. First, Amy suggests that a woman discuss reconstruction with her breast surgeon and have him contact a plastic surgeon to discuss the details of her case. This, if possible, should be done premastectomy. If there are psychological or other factors preventing this preoperative discussion, then a two-stage procedure should be requested to give the woman time to organize that aspect of her thinking.

One of Amy's patients had rushed into reconstruction as soon as possible and then reported that she still had to deal with the reality of having had cancer when it was all over. Reconstruction did not negate a period of mourning. Amy reports that she has yet to come across any woman who regrets having gone through reconstruction even if she has encountered some difficulty with it. Most of the time, she says, women are more concerned with losing their lives than losing their breasts, but occasionally it's different. One woman never mentioned cancer during the entire time she was in the hospital. She was on the phone constantly with her surgeon and her plastic surgeon about whether they could save the nipple. But later, during a visit to Amy, she confessed, "You know, I'm just now beginning to realize that I had cancer." With most women, once a clear pathology report comes through, Amy notes that the breast becomes the big issue. She smiled. "I've noticed that some women consider it a gift to get breasts that they've always wanted when they were never too pleased with their first pair." We parted, and as I walked out into the cold night air, I wished that there had been an Amy to help me through my siege. I would have felt much less lonely.

At Memorial Sloan-Kettering Hospital, Mary Ellen Bowles, C.S.W. (certified social worker), of the Department of Rehabilition, and nurse Annette Beiringer talked with me about their experiences with the inpatient postmastectomy program. We sat in Mary Ellen's tiny office and discussed their concerns about helping the women, a task to which these two gentle people seemed totally dedicated. I had just spent two mornings behind a one-way mirror in an observation room watching Mary Ellen and Annette lead a group of robed patients through one and a half hours of rehabilitation excercises and group discussion. On the first day Annette announced to the women that a woman writer was present in the observation room. As they all looked toward the mirror, I "scrunched" down in my seat, feeling like a voyeur, but, after that momentary awareness they seemed to forget that I was there. One woman even frequently peered into the mirror to check her hair and makeup. Attending the sessions is included in the doctors' orders for the patients, the aim being physical and emotional rehabilitation as soon after surgery as possible. The topic of reconstruction was brought up almost immediately even though most of the women still appeared traumatized by the mastectomy, one having had a bilateral procedure. I wondered if the look of shock on their faces is the same for all postsurgical patients, or is it particularly vivid with mastectomized women?

I found the group to be an excellent example of "bonding" because of the sharing of reactions. It seemed to break down the feelings of isolation and loneliness. Mary Ellen told me that many women continue their contact when they leave the hospital, some even going through the reconstruction together.

A pretty floor nurse, Angela, came in to demonstrate and pass around various types of external prostheses. She asked if the women had looked at their mastectomy scars. Only one had done so. The others expressed their fear that the scar would be ugly and upsetting. Angela encouraged them to look at it before going home, advising them to call a nurse if they were reluctant to look at the scar alone. The reaction of the women to the prostheses ranged from apathy to nose-wrinkling disgust, some commenting, "It's so heavy . . . it's going to be hot in the summer," and so on.

At the second session I observed, the two main worries expressed were fear of recurrence and missing the breast. One woman said, "I keep forgetting that there's nothing left there to protect." An attractive Reach to Recovery volunteer who had had reconstruction joined the group. She pointed out that both of these concerns were lessened for her by reconstruction; that this had made it all easier to endure. She commented that her husband feels good about reconstruction, because it has made her feel so much better. One patient with liver as well as breast cancer said that she felt less devastated by the recent development of the liver disease than by the breast removal, even though she recognized the irrationality of her reaction.

The group, led by Mary Ellen, made several important points regarding reconstruction:

1. Constant worry about recurrence is a bleak existence. Reconstruction eliminates the visual reminder, so you can put that worry further away.
2. Reconstruction removes the disease from other people's minds, too. They picture you with breasts, as before.
3. Nobody can tell you what you should do or feel regarding your own body. They can only tell you how *they* feel about what you do. (In this instance, I was reminded of Reach to Recovery's Sue Lucas telling me that she receives occasional calls from husbands requesting reconstruction information for their wives. One husband wanted to cheer his seriously depressed wife with the option of reconstruction, even though he felt it was not important to him. It turned out, though, upon Sue's investigation, that the woman was not at all interested in reconstructing the breast at that point; she was dealing with the confrontation with her own mortality.)

4. If you're mourning the loss, then you owe it to yourself to investigate the option of reconstruction whether you choose it or not.
5. As you get further away from the disease aspect, you become more concerned with the secondary issue, the breast loss. Everyone's timetable is different.

Mary Ellen added that the rehabilitation department at Memorial is available for consultation after discharge. Follow-up workshops, including those on reconstruction, are held every few months. As I sat in Mary Ellen's office, warmed by her and Annette's involvement with the progress of those women, I realized that team effort like theirs is very rare. In most cases, women are isolated after mastectomies in hospitals and communities that have neither the funds nor the organization to provide the much-needed support and information.

9
Help: How and Where to Get It

In 1983, after publishing an article on breast reconstruction in *Woman's Day* magazine, I received a letter that made me realize how fortunate I was to live in an area where information on reconstruction was so readily available. The letter read, in part: "To me, the article expresses some of the same things I was feeling but afraid to express to others. Namely, that having two breasts was very important to me. And, like Marilyn, looking in the mirror was a very big shock. We live in a city of about 150,000 people with an average of 15 mastectomies done each month and yet there is no real place to go to find information on reconstruction."

It's true that information may be more accessible in a major metropolitan area, but no matter where you live or how isolated you feel, there's a lot you can do to help yourself reach a decision about reconstruction. I've put together as many "helping hands" on a national basis as possible. As interest in this topic grows and more and more women become informed enough to investigate it, the list should grow quickly. Remember, positive action erases anger, and doing something, anything, to help yourself makes you feel less impotent and more in control.

In terms of touching base on a person-to-person level, there are several sources. The American Cancer Society's Reach to Recovery program is still the best known and the most widespread.

Address: Reach to Recovery Reconstruction Program
c/o American Cancer Society, Inc., National Headquarters
777 Third Avenue, New York, N.Y. 10017
Phone: (212) 371-2900

The American Cancer Society has 58 national divisions and over 3,100 regional units. These are listed in the white pages of the telephone directory, or you can call your state division to inquire about the location of the nearest regional unit. The units are designed to cover all of the counties in the United States. The Reach to Recovery breast reconstruction program is available at the patient's request after she leaves the hospital. While she is in the hospital, she must be referred to the program by her doctor. Trained volunteers are provided who have undergone reconstruction themselves. In the fall of 1984 the American Cancer Society's new pamphlet will be made available and will contain essentially the same material shown in their slide presentation on breast reconstruction. It is entitled: "Breast Reconstruction After Mastectomy: It's Your Choice" and will be particularly useful if the slides are not available in all units. It will also be part of the Reach to Recovery packet given to women in the hospital. The telephone number and address of the local American Cancer Society office is provided in that pamphlet. You will then be put in touch with a volunteer who has had reconstruction. That volunteer cannot recommend a plastic surgeon, but the state or local unit of the American Cancer Society will provide names of surgeons performing breast reconstruction. For maximum satisfaction, it would be wise, in viewing the slides or reading the pamphlet, also to have direct access to a Reach to Recovery volunteer. The person-to-person aspect is the program's main strength.

Once contacted, the Reach to Recovery volunteer will set

up an appointment for a personal visit. There is no patient cost involved, nor is a commitment to breast reconstruction expected, but the visit can provide much useful information on a one-to-one basis.

Some states have not yet developed the reconstruction visitation program, but a call to the nearest Cancer Society office will provide that information. Interestingly enough, Alaska and Hawaii are two states that do have the program now.

Dr. Diane Fink, a vice-president of the American Cancer Society, observed that women who one year ago would not have considered reconstruction are now interested. When we talked about how mastectomy affects a relationship, she said that, in her experience, if the relationship with a partner is good before cancer, it usually survives.

I spoke to Melvin Wiesenthal, who has been an active Reach to Recovery volunteer for the past five years, dealing with the husbands and partners of mastectomized women. He told me that reconstruction has never come up in his conversations with these men. They seem to be totally focused on the woman's physical and emotional welfare at that point. He acknowledged, however, that his aid was usually enlisted immediately postmastectomy when the emphasis was primarily the confrontation with disease.

I also interviewed several women in various parts of the country who are division coordinators and multistate representatives in the society's reconstruction program. One such source confirmed that many surgeons are still not introducing the topic and quoted the recent remark of an older, conservative physician in her area who, when questioned about informed consent for breast surgery, said, "Women don't need to know anything about their breasts except what size bra to wear." With that in mind, I urge you to be prepared to take the initiative yourself in terms of reconstruction. If your surgeon is encouraging, all the better; it would certainly make your life a bit easier. If not, start making a few phone calls yourself.

CHARTERED DIVISIONS OF THE AMERICAN CANCER SOCIETY

Alabama Division, Inc.
2926 Central Avenue
Birmingham, Alabama 35209
(205) 879-2242

Alaska Division, Inc.
1343 G Street
Anchorage, Alaska 99501
(907) 277-8696

Arizona Division, Inc.
634 West Indian School Road
P.O. Box 33187
Phoenix, Arizona 85067
(602) 234-3266

Arkansas Division, Inc.
5520 West Markham Street
P.O. Box 3822
Little Rock, Arkansas 72203
(501) 664-3480-1-2

California Division, Inc.
1710 Webster Street
P.O. Box 2061
Oakland, California 94612
(415) 893-7900

Colorado Division, Inc.
2255 South Oneida
P.O. Box 24669
Denver, Colorado 80224
(303) 758-2030

Connecticut Division, Inc.
Barnes Park South
14 Village Lane
P.O. Box 410
Wallingford, Connecticut 06492
(203) 265-7161

Delaware Division, Inc.
Academy of Medicine Building
1708 Lovering Avenue
Suite 202
Wilmington, Delaware 19806
(302) 654-6267

District of Columbia Division, Inc.
Universal Building, South
1825 Connecticut Avenue, N.W.
Washington, D.C. 20009
(202) 483-2600

Florida Division, Inc.
1001 South MacDill Avenue
Tampa, Florida 33609
(813) 253-0541

Georgia Division, Inc.
1422 West Peachtree Street, N.W.
Atlanta, Georgia 30309
(404) 892-0026

Hawaii Pacific Division, Inc.
Community Services Center Building
200 North Vineyard Boulevard
Honolulu, Hawaii 96817
(808) 531-1662-3-4-5

Idaho Division, Inc.
1609 Abbs Street
P.O. Box 5386
Boise, Idaho 83705
(208) 343-4609

Illinois Division, Inc.
37 South Wabash Avenue
Chicago, Illinois 60602
(312) 372-0472

Indiana Division, Inc.
4755 Kingsway Drive, Suite 100
Indianapolis, Indiana 46205
(317) 257-5326

Iowa Division, Inc.
Highway #18 West
P.O. Box 980
Mason City, Iowa 50401
(515) 423-0712

Kansas Division, Inc.
3003 Van Buren Street
Topeka, Kansas 66611
(913) 267-0131

Kentucky Division, Inc.
Medical Arts Building
1169 Eastern Parkway
Louisville, Kentucky 40217
(502) 459-1867

Louisiana Division, Inc.
Masonic Temple Building, 7th floor
333 St. Charles Avenue
New Orleans, Louisiana 70130
(504) 523-2029

Maine Division, Inc.
Federal and Green Streets
Brunswick, Maine 04011
(207) 729-3339

Maryland Division, Inc.
200 East Joppa Road
Towson, Maryland 21204
(301) 828-8890

Massachusetts Division, Inc.
247 Commonwealth Avenue
Boston, Massachusetts 02116
(617) 267-2650

Michigan Division, Inc.
1205 East Saginaw Street
Lansing, Michigan 48906
(517) 371-2920

Minnesota Division, Inc.
3316 West 66th Street
Minneapolis, Minnesota 55435
(612) 925-2772

Mississippi Division, Inc.
345 North Mart Plaza
Jackson, Mississippi 39206
(601) 362-8874

Missouri Division, Inc.
3322 American Avenue
P.O. Box 1066
Jefferson City, Missouri 65102
(314) 893-4800

Montana Division, Inc.
2820 First Avenue South
Billings, Montana 59101
(406) 252-7111

Nebraska Division, Inc.
8502 West Center Road
Omaha, Nebraska 68124
(402) 393-5800

Nevada Division, Inc.
1325 East Harmon
Las Vegas, Nevada 89109
(702) 798-6877

New Hampshire Division, Inc.
686 Mast Road
Manchester, New Hampshire 03102
(603) 669-3270

New Jersey Division, Inc.
CN2201, 2600 Route 1
North Brunswick, New Jersey 08902
(201) 297-8000

New Mexico Division, Inc.
5800 Lomas Boulevard, N.E.
Albuquerque, New Mexico 87110
(505) 262-2336

New York State Division, Inc.
6725 Lyons Street, P.O. Box 7
East Syracuse, New York 13057
(315) 437-7025

 Long Island Division, Inc.
 535 Broad Hollow Road
 Route 110
 Melville, New York 11747
 (516) 420-1111

 New York City Division, Inc.
 19 West 56th Street
 New York, New York 10019
 (212) 586-8700

 Queens Division, Inc.
 111-15 Queens Boulevard
 Forest Hills, New York 11375
 (212) 263-2224

 Westchester Division, Inc.
 901 North Broadway
 White Plains, New York 10603
 (914) 949-4800

North Carolina Division, Inc.
222 North Person Street
P.O. Box 27624
Raleigh, North Carolina 27611
(919) 834-8463

North Dakota Division, Inc.
Hotel Graver Annex Building
115 Roberts Street
P.O. Box 426
Fargo, North Dakota 58102
(701) 232-1385

Ohio Division, Inc.
1375 Euclid Avenue
Suite 312
Cleveland, Ohio 44115
(216) 771-6700

Oklahoma Division, Inc.
3800 North Cromwell
Oklahoma City, Oklahoma 73112
(405) 946-5000

Oregon Division, Inc.
0330 S.W. Curry
Portland, Oregon 97201
(503) 295-6422

Pennsylvania Division, Inc.
Route 422 and Sipe Avenue
P.O. Box 416
Hershey, Pennsylvania 17033
(717) 533-6144

 Philadelphia Division, Inc.
 21 South 12th Street
 Philadelphia, Pennsylvania 19107
 (215) 665-2900

Puerto Rico Division, Inc.
(Avenue Domenech 273
Hato Rey, P.R.)
GPO Box 6004
San Juan, Puerto Rico 00936
(809) 764-2295

Rhode Island Division, Inc.
345 Blackstone Boulevard
Providence, Rhode Island
 02906
(401) 831-6970

South Carolina Division, Inc.
2442 Devine Street
Columbia, South Carolina
 29205
(803) 256-0245

South Dakota Division, Inc.
1025 North Minnesota Avenue
Hillcrest Plaza
Sioux Falls, South Dakota
 57104
(605) 336-0897

Tennessee Division, Inc.
713 Melpark Drive
Nashville, Tennessee 37204
(615) 383-1710

Texas Division, Inc.
3834 Spicewood Springs Road
P.O. Box 9863
Austin, Texas 78766
(512) 345-4560

Utah Division, Inc.
610 East South Temple
Salt Lake City, Utah 84102
(801) 322-0431

Vermont Division, Inc.
13 Loomis Street, Drawer C
Montpelier, Vermont 05602
(802) 223-2348

Virginia Division, Inc.
3218 West Cary Street
P.O. Box 7288
Richmond, Virginia 23221
(804) 359-0208

Washington Division, Inc.
2120 First Avenue North
Seattle, Washington 98109
(206) 283-1152

West Virginia Division, Inc.
Suite 100
240 Capitol Street
Charleston, West Virginia
 25301
(304) 344-3611

Wisconsin Division, Inc.
615 North Sherman Avenue
P.O. Box 8370
Madison, Wisconsin 53708
(608) 249-0487

  Milwaukee Division, Inc.
  11401 West Watertown Plank
   Road
  Wauwatosa, Wisconsin 53226
  (414) 453-4500

Wyoming Division, Inc.
Indian Hills Center
506 Shoshoni
Cheyenne, Wyoming 82009
(307) 638-3331

ASPRS (THE AMERICAN SOCIETY OF PLASTIC AND RECONSTRUCTIVE SURGEONS)

Address: 233 North Michigan Avenue
Suite 1900
Chicago, Illinois 60601
Phone: (312) 856-1818 (ASPRS office)
(312) 856-1834 (referral center)

The second telephone number will give you the twenty-four-hour answering machine of the Plastic Surgeons Referral Center. The polite recorded message requests that you leave your name, address, the type of surgery in which you are interested, and the referral source (magazine article, friend, physician, etc.). Within a couple of weeks you will be sent a list of three board-certified plastic surgeons in your area who perform breast reconstruction. (My suggestion would be to interview all three, if possible; certainly more than just one.) A pamphlet on breast reconstruction is sent along with the referrals. Included in this pamphlet is advice for patients who are unable to pay the full surgical fee or even a reduced fee. There is a list of hospitals that offer such surgery at greatly reduced rates. Included are university and teaching hospitals, government-run hospitals, and hospitals with plastic surgery training programs. For further help in this area, write to ASPRS.

TEL-MED

In most cities, this service is listed in the white pages of the telephone directory and provides a series of audiotapes. Request the tape on breast reconstruction. If you cannot find a local listing, your doctor's office should be able to provide information about the nearest Tel-Med.

THE SURGICAL OPINION HOTLINE

The National Second Surgical Opinion Program operates a toll-free telephone hot line to help you find a surgeon in your area for a second opinion.
National number: 1-800-638-6833
For Maryland only: 1-800-492-6603

MORE TIPS ON REFERRALS

First, try talking to your cancer surgeon or your family doctor about a referral to a plastic surgeon. You can also call the nearest teaching hospital (one affiliated with a medical school) for names of plastic surgeons. Interview more than one, asking for explanations of their techniques for breast reconstruction.

Your local medical society will provide a list of doctors and their specialties. Remember, it is better to take the recommendation of another professional rather than that of a friend. The friend can tell you about the doctor's "bedside manner" but cannot thoroughly evaluate his or her surgical expertise. A layman's (in this case, laywoman's) advice is not to be discounted, however; e.g., was she pleased with the results, treatment, etc.?

RENU

Address: P.O. Box 8852
          Elkins Park, Pennsylvania 19117
Hot line: (215) 635-1499
Other active RENU programs, in Cleveland and Washington, D.C., are affiliated with the American Cancer Society.
Washington number: (202) 483-2600
Cleveland number: (216) 356-2683

RENU is an acronym for Reconstruction Education for National Understanding and is a breast reconstruction counseling service. Based in Philadelphia, with a twenty-four-hour hot line, it is a volunteer support group composed of women who have had mastectomy and reconstruction. I first learned about RENU when I received a letter and brochure from its secretary, Sondra Bennett, in response to my magazine article in *Woman's Day*. I then spent a pleasant day in Philadelphia talking to Barbara German ("hard" *G* as in "girl"), RENU's enthusiastic founder, and chairperson Ellen Greenfield. They told me that RENU is supervised by the medical staff in the Breast Cancer Program at the Albert Einstein Medical Center in Philadelphia. Barbara and Ellen both received intensive training in reconstruction counseling at the Cleveland Clinic, and Barbara, in turn, set up training programs under the supervision of the Philadelphia medical specialists for other volunteers. All of the RENU women must undergo the same type of program before qualifying as peer counselors. As such, they provide nonmedical information and will counsel women facing mastectomy on the reconstructive options. RENU offers an audiovisual presentation designed by Dr. Wendy Shain, who is also responsible for the American Cancer Society's slide presentation on breast reconstruction. Printed material from ASPRS is also available. The counselors are not permitted to make specific surgery referrals but can give advice on how to go about finding a qualified plastic surgeon. The hot line takes calls from those needing help all over the country, as well as from women wishing to become trained volunteers. All calls are returned free of charge, and the cassettes of the slide presentation are available in various regional hospitals. RENU is available to conduct training sessions in other cities, as well as panels on breast reconstruction. Barbara described the average panel as being about one hour in length, plus a question and answer period. The panel is comprised of a RENU volunteer, a breast surgeon, a guest plastic surgeon, a speaker on the surgical alternative of lumpectomy-radiation, a gynecological consultant, and, if possible, an audience member who has had reconstruction. When

I asked Barbara if she and her counselors were ready and willing to visit any part of the country for training and panels, she smiled broadly and said, "Why not? our motto is Have Reconstruction, Will Travel."

ENCORE

Address: Encore Supervisor
National Board YWCA
135 West 50th Street
New York, New York 10020
Phone: (212) 621-5115

Patricia Hogan, Ph.D., has a business card that reads: "Health, Physical Education, and Recreation Consultant" for the YWCA. Part of her job is to supervise Encore, the Discussion and Exercise Program for Women Who Have Had Breast Cancer Surgery. There are ninety Encore programs around the country. To find the "Y" closest to you with an Encore program, write or call the New York YWCA office. Dr. Hogan suggests that you also request that your local "Y" incorporate the program if it isn't already offered. She described it as primarily an exercise and discussion program, but the group members dictate the choice of topics and the subject of reconstruction is addressed when requested. There is also a manual with a section on breast reconstruction. The sessions are held once a week and are ninety minutes in length, divided into three sections: floor exercise, pool exercise, and discussion. Doctors and technicians are brought in periodically to speak on related topics. Dr. Hogan emphasized that special training in the areas of health and physical education is mandatory for the Encore professional, who must also undergo an intensive workshop in postmastectomy rehabilitation. The program's greatest strength, she feels, is that it provides support and networking for women who are feeling isolated. YWCA membership is waived for Encore participants, and the fee for the course is very low: $10.00 for eight classes, $2.00 per single session. Dr. Hogan says, "We try to make sure that no one is excluded from help for lack of funds."

SHARE

Address: SHARE, c/o Blanche Green
34 Gramercy Park
New York, New York 10003
Hot line: (212) 228-3064 (Answering machine with personal response within twenty-four hours)

SHARE is a shorter way of identifying the Self-Help and Rap Experience for Individuals Who Have Breast Disease/Cancer. Established in 1976 by Dr. Eugene Thiessen, a breast specialist, the New York–based organization provides support for women wishing to share in the discussion of all aspects of breast disease—a peer support group. Special programs are held on specific topics such as chemotherapy, sexuality, nutrition, and reconstruction. The cost of returning the hot-line calls is often assumed by the volunteer making the call, but occasionally, the machine's message advises, the return call may have to be collect. Meetings are held in New York City, but the hot line is, of course, nationally accessible. Volunteers are trained for the hot line and there are certified social workers on the board of directors. They do not provide therapy or formal counseling. Money is raised by donations and a $10.00 membership fee. Membership is not limited to women who have had breast cancer or breast disease, although the majority have. Several members have undergone reconstruction and are able to counsel those women interested. If you call the hot line for information on reconstruction, specify that in your message. The group provides a pamphlet on reconstruction written by Rita Meyer, a member. Dr. Thiessen having moved out of state, there is no direct medical supervision available to SHARE at present. The group does, however, have direct access to the library at the Center for Medical Consumers, which affords a considerable amount of material on all aspects of breast disease and reconstruction.

I spoke at length with social worker and SHARE board member Jackie Feldstein. Her experience has been that women who would go through all the necessary research for reconstruction would do the same for anything. "An ostrich will still be an ostrich. Some women blame everything in their lives on mastectomy without recognizing that it was all there before. If they divorce, many times the marriages were already in trouble." Jackie is afraid that the fantasy level can be dangerous with reconstruction, i.e., "This is going to make me just like I was before." She sees more women now aware of the possibility of reconstruction, asking more questions in group discussions. Very often, however, women don't even know the questions to ask. She advises them to do research first, saying, "If you don't know the questions, you're not going to get the answers."

Diane George, along with Rita Meyer, heads the rap groups at SHARE dealing with reconstruction. She told me that she has spoken to many women who refuse to date at all after mastectomy, whereas the reconstructed women are happy even with complications. She has observed that the women who are violently opposed to reconstruction are those whose problems are the same ones they had before mastectomy—only now they're magnified. Diane says, "They just add mastectomy to their list of things to be angry about." She enumerated the common fears expressed regarding reconstruction:

1. The fear that it won't be a "perfect" result.
2. The fear of undergoing more surgery.
3. The fear of cancer showing up again in surgery.
4. The fear of having anything more done to their breasts.
5. The fear of interfering with some regained sensation on the mastectomized side.

Diane cautions the women that reconstruction will not make the cancer experience disappear, and that if a man is squeamish about cancer, an implant will not alter that. To illustrate the acceptance of mastectomy, she cited the example of a friend, a longtime nudist, who, even though it took her a while, still practices group nudism without a reconstruction.

One cold, rainy Sunday afternoon I joined about twenty women in a church basement for a SHARE meeting. As a result I realized that, even though medical supervision is indeed a vital and necessary factor in dispelling the myths that can be passed on by laypersons with many questions and little medical knowledge, there is something very special indeed about the kind of comfort that a peer group like SHARE affords a breast cancer veteran. An indication of that was the letter read by Jackie Feldstein at the opening of the meeting. It said, in part: "I cannot stress too much the feeling of walking into the first SHARE meeting and knowing that every woman there had had this experience also. For the first time in five years, I was with a group of my peers, at least as related to this one very important aspect of my experience. In a room full of strangers, I felt immediate kinship, acceptance, and enormous potential for sharing experiences with a group of women, different enough from me to provide experiences with which I could compare and measure. The very first five minutes of being in this roomful of women made me feel less isolated. Through sharing with them, all these women who were open enough and brave enough to have chosen this route to self-help, I was able to achieve a much higher level of self-acceptance and even self-love. . . . It is sometimes painful to experience the pain of others but, yet, the good will for me outweighed those negatives." As Jackie Feldstein observed, "SHARE has helped a lot of women to learn to share in their medical treatment, to be not just recipients but participants."

CHUMS

New York address: 3310 Rochambeau Avenue
                  Bronx, New York 10467
Phone: (212) 655-7566

Dr. Sarah Splaver, a clinical psychologist, is the enthusiastic founder and president of CHUMS (Cancer Hopefuls United for Mutual Support), started in September, 1981. The New York–based organization, an outgrowth of the Breast Disease Association of America (BDAA), reports a Nationwide Crisis Intervention and Information Service, Phone-a-Patient and Visit-a-Patient programs, as well as a Pen Pal program to correspond with someone who has the same form of cancer. All forms of cancer are dealt with. Frequent guest speakers, experts in various fields, deliver talks on related topics, breast reconstruction among them. Women interested in breast reconstruction are put in touch with others who either have had the surgery or are investigating it. The tax-deductible annual membership is $10.00. A newsletter reports the encouraging gains in the medical field regarding cancer detection and treatment, as well as the current survival statistics ("More than 3 million people in the United States are alive with a history of cancer and over 2 million of those are five and more years past diagnosis").

To qualify as the head of a CHUMS chapter, the individual must adhere to very firm guidelines espousing only conventional medical treatments. Extensive questionnaires and interviews are part of the selection procedure. Instruction is offered on how to start and lead a new chapter. Most of the chapter heads are trained in nursing, psychology, or rehabilitation.

One bitter cold February afternoon I attended a CHUMS meeting at the American Cancer Society's New York Chapter offices. Approximately forty people gathered in a large ground-floor lounge overlooking a sunlit garden. I paid $5.00 on entry and received, in exchange, several pamphlets describing CHUMS and its philosophy ("Cancer VICTORS, not victims; HOPEFULS, not hopeless"), a hand-crocheted turquoise bookmark, a tiny volume of poetry written by Dr. Splaver during her treatment for breast cancer, a plastic Citibank key ring, and a raffle ticket, #248.

I was greeted by Dr. Splaver, a cross between my Aunt Sadye and Mrs. Santa Claus. About five feet tall, she sported short graying hair and bright red lipstick. Dressed in a cherry red pants suit, tight waistband circling a generous waistline, pants tucked into high boots, she "worked" the room with more energy than I thought possible in one small person. Sarah's remarkably accurate portrait, done by the "in-house" caricaturist Arnold Bergere, bore her quote: "Heck, I'm not afraid of cancer! Cancer's afraid of me!" The caricaturist's $10.00 fee is tax-deductible and was turned back to CHUMS, as was the fee for the readings of Frederick Davies, the "resident" astrologer–card reader. Both men were present at the meeting and donated their services to the organization. A long buffet table was laid with a generous assortment of salads, pastries, and beverages.

The first half of the meeting was devoted to mixing with the group, men and women of all ages with cancer experiences in common. I spoke to one attractive, youngish woman who wore a CHUMS ribbon across her chest, indicating that she was a hostess. Her husband, not she, was the cancer patient, but he was not present that day. "He's handling it very well," she explained. "I'm here because I'm the one who needs the help with it. As a patient and a patient's family, you feel you have a friend in Sarah. She knows everyone by their first name, and you always leave feeling stronger than when you arrived."

The second half of the meeting was an informal rap session headed by Sarah, with members contributing encouraging reports and raising questions about treatment and rehabilitation. For the first time in my life, I won a door prize (one of many), a paperback copy of Bruno Bettelheim's *Freud and Man's Soul.* One newcomer, a tiny miniskirted black girl, got a laugh from all present as she collected her prize, *Bodybuilding for Women.*

Sarah is a firm believer that you can bolster your immune

system by being emotionally and psychologically supportive. At the end of the session, as she told me of CHUMS' activities, several members approached her to say that even though they had been depressed when they arrived, they felt remarkably reassured and uplifted after the meeting. They seemed to feel more convinced than ever of their ability to rehabilitate themselves and put the cancer experience behind them. From what I observed that day, the level of mutual aid was extremely high at CHUMS.

Other Chapters of CHUMS:

San Fernando Valley and Greater Los Angeles Chapter
Chapter Head: LaVerne Fisher, R.N.
13941 Stroud Street
Van Nuys, California 91402
(818) 785-8086

Palm Beach County Chapter
Chapter Head: Sheila C. Furr, Ph.D.
5258 Linton Boulevard (304)
Delray Beach, Florida 33445
(305) 499-5900

Central Maine Chapter
Chapter Head: Mary S. Kinney
RFD 1, Box 8125
Waterville, Maine 04901
(207) 465-7007

Sanford, Maine, and Environs Chapter
Chapter Head: Nina M. Chabot
11 East Street
Sanford, Maine 04073
(207) 324-2843

Maryland, Washington, D.C., Chapter
Chapter Head: Mary Hull Levyne
12189 Mount Albert Road
Ellicott City, Maryland 21043
(301) 531-5949

Monmouth County/South Shore Chapter
Chapter Head: Patty Robbins
518 Warren Avenue
Spring Lake, New Jersey 07762
(201) 449-3149

Mohawk Valley Chapter
Chapter Head: Gerald Levin
R.F.D. Country Club Road
Herkimer, New York 13350
(315) 866-1234

Greater Charlotte Chapter
Chapter Head: Valdaree W. Shull, Ph.D.
1312 Wesson Road
Shelby, North Carolina 28150
(704) 487-8421

Pittsburgh Chapter
Chapter Head: Maureen
  McKenna Mays
309 Meadow Street
Cheswick, Pennsylvania 15024
(412) 274-5592

Knoxville/Oakridge Chapter
Chapter Head: J. Paul Blakely
9635 Tunbridge Lane
Knoxville, Tennessee 37922
(615) 693-1594

Fox Valley Wisconsin Chapter
Chapter Head: Carol S. Krenke
619 West Ninth Avenue
Oshkosh, Wisconsin 54901
(414) 231-7713

RESEARCH THROUGH READING

Reading as much as possible about the current "state of the art" of breast reconstruction can help you to make a thoroughly informed decision. This reading material includes not only periodicals, books, and special magazine articles, but your insurance policies as well—anything and everything to fill in the gaps between mastectomy and peace of mind.

The National Cancer Institute (NCI)

Address: Office of Cancer Communications
          NCI
          Bethesda, Maryland 20205
Telephone for the Cancer Information Service:
          1-800-4-CANCER
Additional numbers:
          1-800-638-6070 (Alaska)
          (202) 635-5700 (Washington, D.C., and suburbs)
          (808) 524-1234 (Oahu; call collect from neighboring
          Hawaiian islands)
Spanish-speaking staff members are available during the daytime hours to those calling from the following areas: California (area codes 213, 714, 619, and 805), Florida, Georgia, Illinois, Northern New Jersey, New York City, and Texas.

The Cancer Information Service (CIS) is a toll-free telephone program sponsored by the National Cancer Institute. It is available nationwide, and your call will be answered by a trained information specialist on reconstruction.

NCI also publishes a booklet on breast reconstruction entitled *Breast Reconstruction: A Matter of Choice*, as well as a chapter on breast reconstruction in their *Breast Cancer Digest*.

Many medical libraries will now open their doors to medical consumers, but several cities also have libraries to answer the specific needs of medical consumers, the laypersons wishing to educate themselves better to medical issues and treatment options. Following is a list and description of several such centers around the country. A word of advice: make sure that you obtain the most recently published articles and statistics when using any library facility. The field of breast cancer surgery and reconstruction is changing rapidly, and you will want to have the very latest information in terms of making your decision. Most public libraries also contain the Directory of Medical Specialists, which provides a listing of all board-certified physicians according to their specialty.

The Center for Medical Consumers

Director: Arthur A. Levin, M.P.H.
Address: 239 Thompson Street
         New York, New York 10012
Phone: (212) 674-7105

The library at the Center for Medical Consumers serves a useful purpose for people who have to make treatment decisions. There is a generous assortment of articles and books relating to breast cancer and reconstruction.

Health Facts is a monthly publication, a consumer newsletter providing information on medical practices and nonmedical alternatives. It covers a broad range of topics, breast cancer and reconstruction among them. Subscriptions are available through the center at the above address. Annual subscription rates are $18.00, each issue being $2.25.

The center has also published a guide, *Your Rights to Your Medical Records; Your Rights as a Hospital Patient.* It contains a state-by-state chart showing variations in the laws covering access to medical records and specific advice on how to go about obtaining your medical records and protecting your rights.

Planetree Health Resource Center

Director: Patricia Phelan
Address: 2040 Webster Street
San Francisco, California 94115
Phone: (415) 346-4636

Planetree is a medical library for the public. It is affiliated with Pacific Medical Center, which has a full medical library on which to draw. Planetree's collection is independently funded and autonomous, however. Planetree's director, Patricia Phelan, told me that the center also offers a research service by mail. Send a cover letter explaining your specific area of interest, and, for $5.00, very basic information on a common health topic will be provided. For $35.00 you can receive a large in-depth study involving a computer search and abstracts of all up-to-date articles. Allow two weeks for the research. In a May 1983 *Ms.* magazine article by Donna Ruscavage ("How to Be Your Own Second Opinion: A Guide to Medical Consumers"), Ms. Phelan is quoted as saying: "The aim of Planetree users isn't to reject medical advice; they simply want to be able to return to their doctors and ask intelligent questions about their conditions."

Consumer Health Information Center

Director: Julie O'Brien
Address: 680 East 600 South
Salt Lake City, Utah 84102
Phone: (801) 364-9318

Located in an old Victorian house and affiliated with Latter Day Saints (LDS) Hospital, this facility makes the University of Utah Library available to center users. Visitors are encouraged, but the center also provides a computer mail search for $5.00 plus mail charges and the pamphlet purchase price. Write requesting information on a specific topic.

Health Education Center

Director: Lois Michaels
Address: 200 Ross Street
Pittsburgh, Pennsylvania 15219
Phone: (412) 392-3160

This medical consumer facility offers a Tel-Aid system featuring many tapes on a variety of medical issues. The center is described as functioning as an interpreter between the layperson and the medical professional.

National Women's Health Network

Address: 224 Seventh Street S.E.
Washington, D.C. 20003
Phone: (202) 543-9222

This is a clearinghouse for literature on women's health issues that will provide pamphlets, printouts, and recommendations for reading on breast reconstruction. There is, occasionally, a minimal copying charge. The network also offers a bimonthly newsletter.

The Patient's Medical Library

Address: 20 Hospital Drive
Toms River, New Jersey 08753
Toll-free number: 1-800-222-0077

This is a group of over forty health researchers who, for a $10.00 fee, will send you the current literature on any medical issue, including research, drug information, medical options, and explanations of medical terminology.

INSURANCE: COSTS AND COVERAGE

Reconstructive surgery is generally more costly than mastectomy, with widely variable fees. In an informal survey conducted in 1982 by the National Cancer Institute, fees ranged from $500 to $5,000. The fees depend upon the type and extent of surgery, the area of the country, and the individual surgeon. Costs are considerably higher, for example, in New York City and Los Angeles, but insurance companies do take that factor into consideration when calculating reimbursement. For a simple implantation, the fees in 1982 ranged from $800 to $3,000, with the average being $1,000. At that time the cost for the more extensive latissimus dorsi operation ranged from $1,000 to $4,000, with an average of $2,000. Nipple-areola graft costs varied between $500 and $1,500 with a typical charge of $700. In 1984 the top fee recorded for the same procedure is $2,500. Costs of all of the procedures have kept pace with inflation. In an informal 1984 survey of fifteen plastic surgeons representing a national geographic distribution, a spokeswoman for the ASPRS reports a range of reconstruction fees from $1,500 to $4,500. This group did not include New York or Los Angeles figures, which tend to pull the average way up ($6,000 is not uncommon in New York for a simple implantation with a nipple-areola graft). Among the fifteen surgeons polled, the range of fees for simple implantation alone was $1,500 to $2,500 with the costs for tissue expanders and flap procedures reaching up to $4,500. In bilateral reconstruction, simple implantation was in the $2,500 range. In 1984, my own inquiry into the gluteal flap procedure produced a range of $5,000 to $6,000, dependent upon the individual case. The ASPRS also reports a range today of from $1,500 to $3,000 for a subcutaneous mastectomy-implant procedure. This is when the breast tissue is removed leaving the outer skin and nipple intact. The implant is then inserted to compensate for the tissue loss.

As in all operative procedures, extra expenses are hospitalization costs, operating room, and anesthesia charges. Most plastic surgeons request payment in advance. The patient is then reimbursed by her insurance company. A letter and a description of the procedure from the surgeon to the company will determine in advance of surgery the amount of reimbursement. However, pre-authorization does not mean that the company will pay before surgery. The patient is still reimbursed after she has paid the surgeon. I spoke to several women who had obtained personal or bank loans to finance their reconstruction until they could be reimbursed by their insurance companies.

When breast reconstruction was in its infancy, insurance companies refused reimbursement on the basis of its being labelled "cosmetic" surgery. That has changed, happily, and it is now included under the heading of rehabilitative surgery by most companies. Dr. Randolph Guthrie's secretary reports that if companies balk at payment for reconstruction, she just sends them a copy of the ruling of the Insurance Department of the State of New York that states that cosmetic surgery will not be covered "EXCEPT that 'cosmetic surgery' shall NOT INCLUDE reconstructive surgery resulting from trauma, infection, or other DISEASES of the involved part." She says that payment always follows. She reports very poor reimbursement with just Blue Cross/Blue Shield and also with GHI (Group Health Insurance) and tells me that very seldom will any company commit itself to a specific sum in advance. Surgery on the opposite breast, she says, usually requires a letter or two from the surgeon describing the rehabilitative necessity of the procedure. It's simpler, reimbursement-wise, if any matching surgery on the opposite breast is done at the same time as the reconstruction.

I called Blue Cross/Blue Shield in Los Angeles, without identifying myself, and told them that I was about to undergo breast reconstruction. I asked what I could expect in the way of reimbursement and was told that, with Major Medical as well, they would pay 100 percent of a semiprivate or equivalent hospital room, 80 percent of the anesthesia charge, and 80 percent for the surgical assistant. As for the surgeon's fee, I was advised to have him write a description of what he planned to do (including the standard descriptive code numbers used to identify procedures). That would then make it possible for the company to give a preauthorization for payment. Also, if surgery were required on the second breast to achieve a "match," the surgeon was advised to describe that as a "functional problem."

When I called the New York office of Blue Cross/Blue Shield and told the woman I talked to of my anticipated surgery, her reply was, "Uh oh, breast reconstruction! We have a very limited policy on that." She explained that, with Major Medical added to Blue Cross/Blue Shield, however, I would receive 80 percent of a "reasonable and customary" surgical fee. That is determined by the standard range of fees in the specific area in which the surgery is performed.

Major Medical is designed to supplement the basic coverage provided by Blue Cross/Blue Shield. The latter provide their own form of Major Medical supplement, as do most commercial carriers. Medicare is designed for those over sixty-five and is a nationwide program administered state by state. Medicaid is for those who are medically indigent and is state-administered. Insurance regulations can vary, however, from state to state.

My advice to all women would be to avoid any potential difficulty by careful examination of your insurance coverage in this area, "just in case." Forewarned is forearmed and all that. . . . It can make a tremendous difference if the need for breast reconstruction presents itself, and many companies now offer very adequate coverage. Question your insurance agent about what your coverage would be in terms of hospital stay, surgical fee, and number of procedures required. With more women demanding reconstruction, even the most reluctant companies, as well as the government plans for clinic patients, will, I hope, be pressured into broadening their coverage and increasing their allotments. Insurance is, after all, supposed to be a service industry answering the communal need. One woman in her seventies told me that her insurance company paid 93 percent of her total claim for breast reconstruction after she wrote a personal letter telling it what the operation meant to the quality of her life. So keep that in mind, too.

10
Questions for the Plastic Surgeon

Your research into reconstruction can be done anytime: before mastectomy, immediately after, or years later. If you are considering immediate reconstruction, obviously you will want to settle that issue before you go in for surgery. In any case, it helps to do some, if not all, of your research in advance of surgery, since it provides a positive outlet for all of the emotional energy you're generating. It also gives you a much needed sense of control and focuses on the positive aspect of the experience. Some women may feel that they are too emotional at this time to concentrate on the details of rebuilding the breast. In that case, there is no harm done in putting it off until you're feeling more emotionally stable. Just having the option of saying yes or no to reconstruction is an enormously helpful thought to keep in the back of your mind.

If you are not opting for immediate reconstruction for a variety of reasons, tell your breast surgeon that you are interested in breast reconstruction and ask that he (or she) keep that in mind in terms of incision. Obviously, he should remove what he must to ensure the eradication of the disease, but the incision placement may be one choice he can make without jeopardizing his goal and still enable the plastic surgeon to produce the best cosmetic result. The plastic surgeon may even be amenable to consulting with your breast surgeon before or after mastectomy to better acquaint himself with the details of your case.

Once your breast surgeon has given you the green light in terms of breast reconstruction, here is a list of questions for the plastic surgeons you interview. Take it along with you and jot down your notes on a pad. You can even take along a little tape recorder so you can more easily digest his answers a second time at home. Whether you are investigating immediate or delayed reconstruction, most of these questions will apply to either case. Select those appropriate to you. Exact predictions by the surgeon are difficult to make, since each case/body is different, but general guidelines can be given. It may be disconcerting to hear, but this field is an art, not an exact science. It's important to be very frank with the surgeon. Tell him your fantasy of the perfect breasts for you. That's the only way he will know if he can help you realize or approximate your concept. If you are dissatisfied after reconstruction, you must discuss that openly with the surgeon as well. Don't fall into that old "martyr" trap of "If he really cared, he'd know my needs without my having to tell him." That old saw doesn't work in any relationship, so why expect it to work here?

A previsit call to the surgeon's office can inform you of his fee for consultation as well as the range of fees for the various reconstructive procedures. It's best to get those details out of the way first, to avoid any misunderstanding later.

1. What percentage of your practice is devoted to breast reconstruction?
2. Do you perform flap procedures as well as implants? Which ones?
3. What type of reconstructive procedure is appropriate for me, and why?
4. Can I have immediate reconstruction?
5. How long will a simultaneous mastectomy-reconstructive procedure take?
6. Will you consult with my breast surgeon about me before reconstruction?

Questions for the Plastic Surgeon

7. Will it help you to have a photo of my breast before mastectomy?
8. If I choose to use an implant and it is appropriate for me, what type do you prefer? Why?
9. What size implant would you suggest using? Can you duplicate the size of the other breast?
10. Can we achieve a "match" without surgery on the opposite breast?
11. Can we reduce/augment the size of my natural breasts? (This is where the fantasy comes in.)
12. May I see the implant? The size?
13. Where do you prefer making the incision for implant insertion, and how long is it?
14. Do you use the mastectomy incision? If not, why?
15. If I need an expander, how is it expanded and how long before the permanent implant can be inserted?
16. If we take transplanted tissue, where do you suggest it come from? Why?
17. If we do a flap reconstruction, will it require an implant as well?
18. If a flap is used, can you describe the extent and location of the donor site scars?
19. How long will the surgery take?
20. What kind of anesthesia will it require? Will I be premedicated before going up to surgery?
21. Where will the postsurgical drain be located and how long does it remain in place? Is the recovery time longer with a flap than with an implant?
22. Will I have pain? For approximately how long?
23. Will I be bandaged when I wake up? How much?
24. Will I lose any more sensation on the mastectomized side than I already have? If so, is it likely to return?
25. How long will I be in the hospital?
26. How long will I recuperate at home before returning to work?
27. Will my physical activity be limited? How much and for how long?
28. What are the complications that can occur with this method and what can be done to correct them? Can cor-

rective procedures be done under local anesthesia on an outpatient basis?
29. What precautions, if any, should I take after surgery to avoid complications?
30. What would you do to the natural breast to achieve the best match? Where would the scar be? Do your patients report sensation loss?
31. If I do not choose to tuck the other breast, will there be a match in a brassiere?
32. If I decided to tuck the other breast, could that be done later, with the nipple-areola grafts?
33. Where will we take the grafts for the nipple-areola complex? (a) Is that an outpatient procedure? (b) How long will it take? (c) What is the cost? (d) How long is the recuperative period? (e) How soon after the first stage can that be done?
34. How often will you want to see me after reconstruction?
35. Will I be able to wear revealing clothes? Strapless dresses? Bathing suits?
36. Will I be comfortable sleeping on my breast?
37. Will there be changes in the appearance of the reconstructed breast six months later? One year later?
38. If tailoring or "touch up" procedures are necessary to achieve the best possible result, is that covered by your basic surgical fee? Also, is any treatment for complications covered?
39. May I see "before and after" photos of these procedures, including the flap donor sites?
40. May I speak to any of your patients who have had breast reconstruction?

Index

Adjuvant chemotherapy, 19, 63
Age differences, 80, 99, 107, 124, 163
Albert Einstein Medical Center, Philadelphia, 61, 177
American Cancer Society, 71, 112, 171-174
American Society for Therapeutic Radiation Oncology (ASTRO), 71
American Society of Plastic and Reconstructive Surgeons (ASPRS), 96, 175, 177, 189-190
Anderson, M.D., Clinic, Houston, 117
Augmentation, 82

Beiringer, Annette, 165
Bennett, Sondra, 177
Bilateral reconstruction, 190
Birnbaum implant, 97
Blue Cross/Blue Shield, 190-191
Bonadonna, Gianni, 34

Bowles, Mary Ellen, 165-167
Breast Cancer Advisory Center, Kensington, Maryland, 71
Breast Cancer Digest, 186
Breast Cancer Symposium, Annual, 70
Breast Disease Association of America (BDAA), 182

Caine, Lynn, 54
Calle, Dr., 66-67
Cancer Information Service (CIS), 186
Capsule, tight, 93-95, 113, 116
Center for Medical Consumers, 180, 186-187
Chaglassian, Ted A., 125
Chemotherapy, 19, 22-23, 59, 63-64, 65-66, 68, 81-82, 99, 118, 122
Chou, Amy, 161-164
CHUMS (Cancer Hopefuls United for Mutual Support), 182-185

Columbia-Presbyterian Medical Center, 61, 64, 100, 115, 117, 124
Consumer Health Information Center, 188
Counseling, 155-156, 158, 165
Curie Institute, Paris, 66
Cytoxan, 23

Denial, 56
Depression, 54, 56, 120-121, 122, 123
DeVito, Robert, 79
Dexon, (sutures), 99
Directory of Medical Specialists, 116
Directory of Professional Social Workers, 155
Donor site, 109, 110-111
  nipple graft, 47-48, 98-99
Double-lumen implants, 92, 96, 112-113, 119
Dow Corning, 92, 94

Elliptical island flap, 91
ENCORE, 178
Exercise, 178
Expanders, 78, 97, 101, 113-114

Fees, 189-190
Feldstein, Jackie, 180, 181
Fink, Diane, 170
Fluorouracil, 23
Freeman, Bromley S., 125
Fujino, Toyomi, 105

George, Diane, 180
German, Barbara, 177
GHI (Group Health Insurance), 190
Gluteal free flap, 78-79, 105, 107, 108-109, 115, 190
Goin, John, 123, 124
Goin, Marcia, 123, 124
Granulocyte count, 64
Green, Blanche, 179
Greenfield, Ellen, 177
Gumport, Stephen L., 159, 160
Guthrie, Randolph, Jr., 82-100, 104

Habif, David, 61-63, 64, 73, 80-81
Halsted radical mastectomy, 57, 78
Harvard Medical School's Joint Center for Radiation Therapy, 64-65
Health Education Center, 188
Health Facts, 186
Hellman, Samuel, 72-74
Hernia (and RAM), 103-104, 109
Heyer-Schulte, 94
Hoffman, Saul, 111-115
Hogan, Patricia, 178
Holland, Jimmie, 125
Holleb, Arthur, 70, 80
"How to Be Your Own Second Opinion," 187
Hugo, Norman, 100-103
Husbands, 158, 166, 170
Hyman, George, 63-64

Implants, 42, 46, 77, 79, 85-97, 105-107, 112-113, 116, 118, 119-120, 189-190
  extrusion of, 87
  infection, 118
  size, 46, 96-97
  subcutaneous, 85, 87
  submuscular, 89, 118
  types, 92
Incision, 81, 88, 112
Infection (implants), 118
Inpatient postmastectomy program, 165
Insurance, health, 72, 82, 92, 155, 189-192
Intraductal carcinoma, 147

Jacobs, Ellen, 125-126

Knoche-Coury Nipple, 103
Kushner, Rose, 71

Latissimus dorsi flap, 42, 78, 79, 91-92, 101, 110, 118, 131, 189
Latter Day Saints Hospital, 188
Leis, Henry, 70-71, 80
Levin, Arthur A., 186
Little, J. W., 86
Lobular neoplasia, 20
Lucas, Sue, 94, 129, 166
Lumpectomy, 59-60, 62-63, 64-65, 67, 69, 72-73
Lymph nodes, 63, 64, 65, 66, 67, 81, 117

McCarthy, Virginia, 160
McGrath, Mary, 117-120
Major Medical, 191
Mammograms, 9
Mammoplasty, 82
Mastectomy, 42, 59-60, 67, 73, 77-79, 190
Mastopexy, 82
Medicaid, 191
Medical Devices Act, 119-120
Medicare, 191
Memorial Sloan-Kettering Cancer Center, 48, 65, 72, 83, 165
Methotrexate, 23
Meyer, Rita, 179
Michaels, Lois, 188
Mount Sinai Hospital, 111
Myocutaneous flap, 118

National Association of Social Workers, 155
National Cancer Institute (NCI), 126, 185-186, 189
National Institutes of Health (NIH), 65-66
National Women's Health Network, 188
Necrosis, 103, 109
New York Hospital, 83, 161
New York Medical College, Valhalla, 70
New York University Medical Center, 70, 104, 156, 158, 159
Nipple-areola graft, 43, 47, 81, 98-100, 109, 113, 119, 131, 189

O'Brien, Julie, 188
Omentum, 43
Oncologist, 22

Parrin, E. R., 95
Partial mastectomy, 59, 69, 73
Partners, 158, 166, 170
Pathology report, 74
Patient's Medical Library, 189
Pectoral muscle, 42, 46, 81, 85, 87-88
Phelan, Patricia, 187
Planetree Health Resource Center, 187
Polyurethane, 93, 95, 120
Prophylactic procedures, 34, 77
Prostheses, 103, 120

Quadrantectomy, 59, 116

Radiation, 59-60, 62-63, 64-65, 66, 67, 68, 70-74, 99, 119
Radiotherapy. See Radiation
Radovan Expander, 114
RAM, 78, 79, 100, 101-102, 103-104, 107, 109-110, 116
Randall, Judith, 120
Reach to Recovery, 129, 164, 169-170
Reconstruction
  contraindications for, 101
  emotional aspect, 106-107, 126
  immediate, 79, 102, 108, 111, 114, 116, 117-118, 119, 121-122, 157
  as lifesaving option, 58-59

Reconstruction Education for National Understanding (RENU), 176-177
Rectus abdominis myodermal flap. See RAM
Rectus muscle, 86, 103-104
Recurrence rates, 34, 65, 67, 69-70, 71, 72-74, 115, 117
Referrals (surgeons), 175-176
Ruscavage, Donna, 187
Rusk, Howard, 156

Saline solution implants, 92, 94, 95, 96, 112
Sawyer, Patricia, 156
Scars, 84-85
Serratus muscle, 85-87
Shain, Wendy, 177
SHARE, 179-181
Shaw, William W., 104-111, 115
Silicone gel implants, 42, 92, 95-96, 105, 106, 107, 112, 116, 119
Sloan-Kettering. See Memorial Sloan-Kettering Cancer Center
Snyderman, Reuven, 83
Somers, Robert, 61, 63, 64, 117-118
Splaver, Sarah, 182, 183-184
Stages (I, II, III), 66-67, 72-73, 117
Steroids, 93, 95, 113, 116
Stevens, Laurie, 117-118, 120-124
Subcutaneous mastectomy, 77, 190
Surgical Opinion Hotline, 176

Survival rates. *See* Recurrence rates
Symonds, Francis, 115-116

Tansini, Ignio, 91
Tel-Aid, 188
Tel-Med, 175
Thiessen, Eugene, 179
Tumorectomy. *See* Lumpectomy

Urban, Jerome, 65-69, 159

Vascular capsule, 93

Washington Post, 120
White cell count, 64
Widow, 54
Wiesenthal, Melvin, 170

Your Rights to Your Medical Records; Your Rights as a Hospital Patient, 187
YWCA, New York, 178
YWHA, Ninety-Second Street, New York City, 160

L R C

100923

362.1 Snyder, Marilyn.
S675i
An informed decision

DATE			

© THE BAKER & TAYLOR CO.